A Practical Guide for Health Professionals

Dr. Shadrick G Lungu

Contents

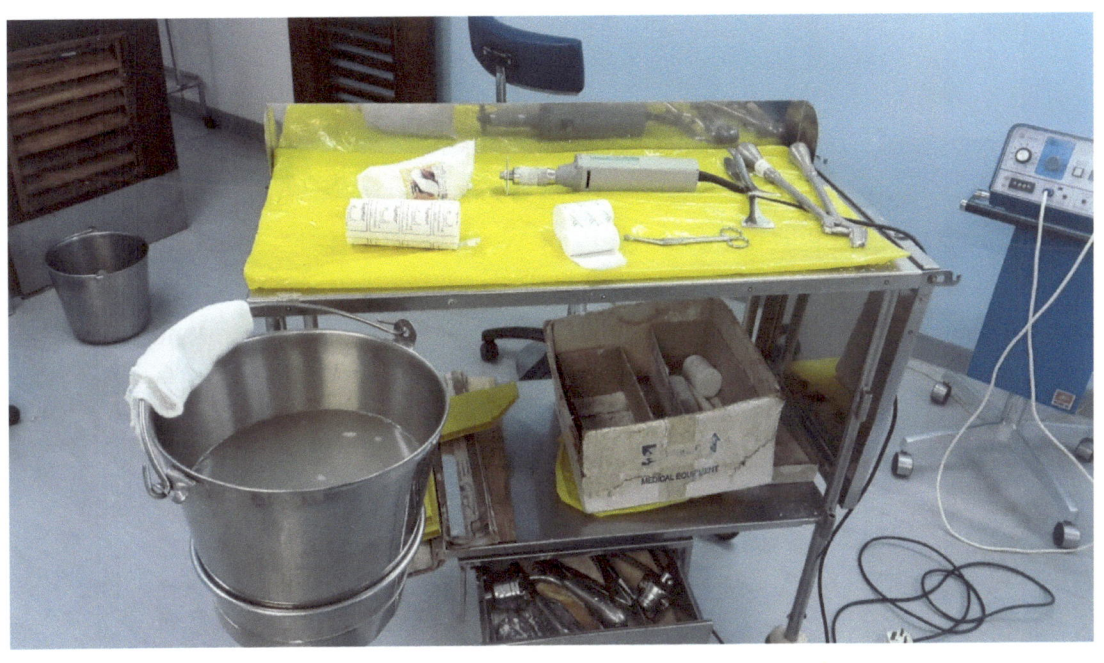

This work is dedicated to my children, Dalitso and Zamiwe; and my wife Martha who, in her own right, is a surgeon. It is my hope that they, too, may draw some inspiration from this gesture (of writing) that they may be able to have the will and power to put their experiences in life into print for the betterment of mankind.

Acknowledgement

I wish to acknowledge Mr. John Banda (a motivational speaker) who, knowingly or unknowingly, planted a seed into me at a Lions District 413 annual convention of July 2013; to start thinking seriously about the potential we all possess – to tell a story and do anything we are passionate about in life. And in this regard, he unleashed and energized my introspection which culminated into the writing on a subject matter that I am truly passionate about, trauma.

I wish to thank my wife Martha for having discovered *CreateSpace* online and therefore wish to offer my profound gratitude and appreciation to *CreateSpace* for having guided me so very well to be able to have this work put together and ultimately published it professionally.

I wish to acknowledge my patients and co-workers (from the hospital and theatre cleaners, nurses and doctors) who provided me with some of the essential materials especially the beautiful pictorial illustrations that have been used in this manual.

I thank all my friends and colleagues that encouraged me to persevere on this journey so that, together, we may see the end product in print!

Last but not the least, I wish to acknowledge the end user of the manual for having chosen to purchase this manual for the wellbeing of our/their patients who are the ultimate consumers and beneficiaries.

Simple and attention to minute detail, are the effective and efficient methods to patient care and are the hallmark and the beginning of looking after mankind...

With the above stated mission statement, this manual is purely borne, designed and written from the practical and teaching experiences of the author in the field of Orthopaedics and Traumatology; having observed the skills and literature gaps in the appropriate medical and health teaching/training materials especially in health institutions, more so, in economically challenged countries like Zambia.

With the foregoing above, the list of references at the end of this work is kept to a bare minimum.

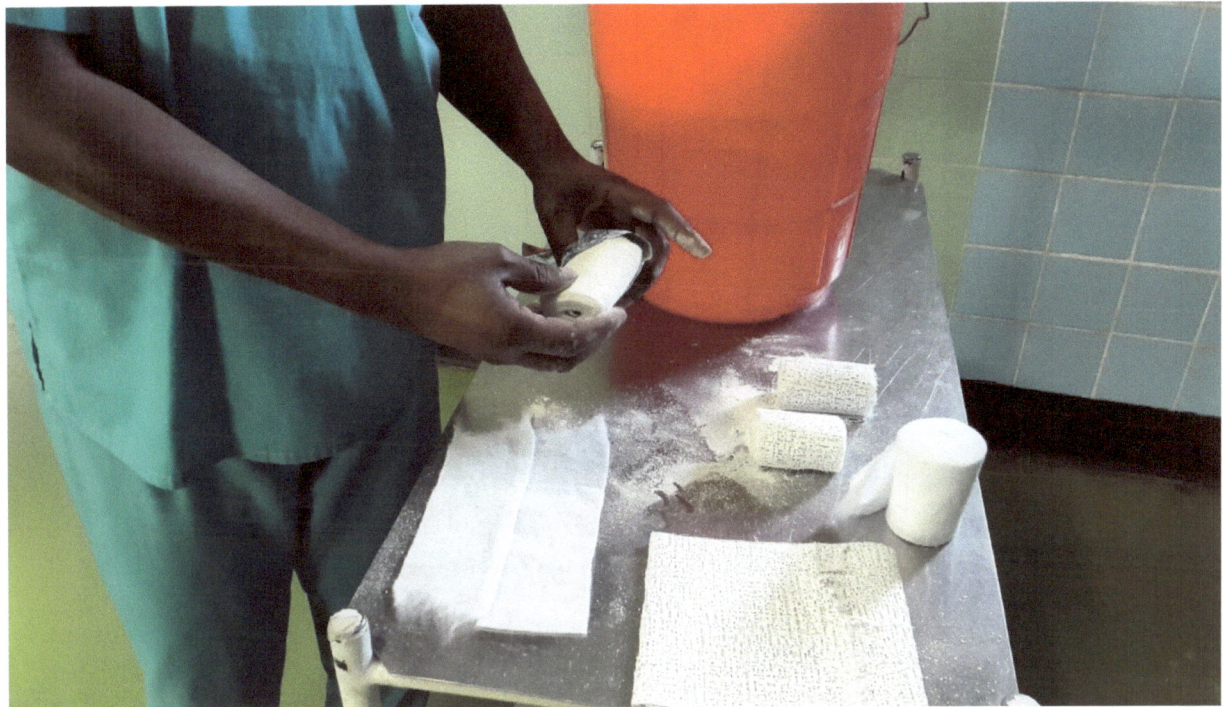

Preparing for a procedure is as important as doing the procedure itself!

Mat   POP bandage   Orthopaedic wool   Electric cutter   Spreader   Manual Shear

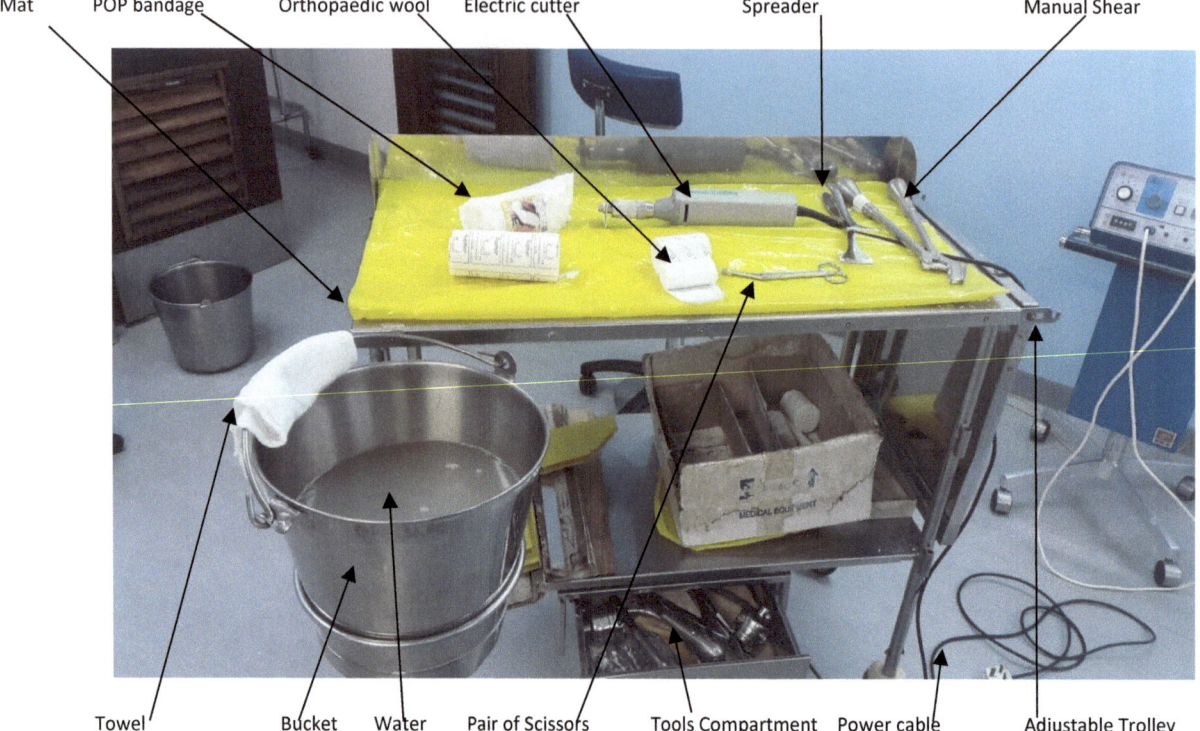

Towel   Bucket   Water   Pair of Scissors   Tools Compartment   Power cable   Adjustable Trolley

Plaster of Paris Trolley

*F*racture management in Zambia has been/is taught in various tertiary health institutions of learning. One of the materials or "tools" used for fracture management in Zambia and, indeed, world over is the Plaster of Paris; commonly known as POP. This is true as observed by Abraham Apley who says "Plaster of Paris is one material that is used widely in fracture management world wide[1]."He also states that "Plaster of Paris can be safe to use. However, in inexperienced hands it can be dangerous[1]." This again tries to emphasize and strengthen the need to drill and educate would be users of Plaster of Paris more diligently and appropriately in its use.

Students, at various levels of their training, learn by:

    a. Simply watching or observing the doctors or whoever is tasked to apply the POP on a patient.
    b. Assisting the doctors applying the POP without active knowledge transfer and while
    c. *A few are actually physically taught how the POP must be applied; in a step by step manner.*

This manual therefore, is written from a background of the author and many others, who had been "trained" in plaster application and techniques, by "osmosis" without a well thought through structured method or system.

The intention and objective of this manual therefore is to put together a simple but, yet, comprehensive structured manual and method of teaching the students and indeed other medical professionals that will deal with non-displaced fractures and indeed other traumatic and non-traumatic conditions requiring the use of Plaster of Paris. It is also intended for the trainers of trainers.

The principles, however, outlined herein can be utilized by, even, qualified General and Orthopaedic surgeons once the displaced fracture is relocated (under anaesthesia) to an acceptable anatomical orientation.

Note: It must be emphasized, however, that this manual is intended for health professionals that will deal with non-displaced fractures.

For a long time, the author of this manual has wondered why this casting bandage or material has been called Plaster of "Paris" and not Plaster of "Lusaka" or any other city.

Gypsum plaster is not a modern invention like Portland cement, as some people might suggest[2]. We know that it was used by the ancient Egyptians to plaster the pyramid at Cheops. In Britain, research being carried out by Claire Gapper, a PhD student at the Courtauld Institute indicates that considerable quantities of Plaster of Paris were being imported from France during Henry VIII's reign for work on royal properties[2].

Our knowledge of the use of gypsum plaster prior to the 19th Century is limited[2].

Plaster of Paris is a calcium sulfate hemi-hydrate: ($CaSO_4$, ½ H_2O) derived from gypsum, a calcium sulfate dihydrate ($CaSO_4$, 2 H_2O), by firing this mineral at relatively low temperature and then reducing it to powder[2].

From Gypsum to Plaster of Paris: Gypsum is a sedimentary rock, which settled through the evaporation of sea water trapped in lagoons. According to the nature of its impurities, gypsum can show various - colors, ranging from white to brown, yellow, gray and pink[2].

The oldest traces of plaster renders are 9,000 years old, and were found in Anatolia and Syria[2]. We also know that 5,000 years ago, the Egyptians burnt gypsum in open-air fires, then crushed it into powder, and finally mixed this powder with water to make jointing material for the blocks of their monuments, such as the magnificent Cheops Pyramid for example. The ancient Egyptians used models of plaster taken directly from the human body[2].

Plaster of Paris: Throughout the centuries, expertise was gained in many parts of the world with gypsum calcinations. In the 1700's, Paris was already the "capital of plaster" ("Plaster of Paris") since all the walls of wooden houses were covered with plaster, as a protection against fire. The King of France had enforced this rule after the big London fire literally destroyed this city in 1666. Large gypsum deposits near Paris have long been mined to manufacture... "Plaster of Paris"[2].

Note: Plaster of Paris can be safe to use. However, in inexperienced hands it can be dangerous[1].

Objectives

The objectives or aims of this manual are:

1. To instruct the reader(s) on a step by step basis on when to apply and what sort of cast to apply on an injured patient (limb) - needing such treatment

2. How to apply the Plaster of Paris (as regards the actual technique)

3. To provide the lecturers (instructors) in various training institutions with a practical guide, or a manual, to effectively deliver not only systematic but also structured lectures to their respective students; in a step-by-step manner

4. To repeat certain aspects in the manual so as to increase the uptake of the materials by the reader

5. Use of pictorial illustrations to help deliver the detail home

Target Groups

In the health care systems, a number of health providers deal with patients with fractures and other Orthopaedic conditions. This manual therefore will not be restricted to the health practitioners in Zambia alone but to anyone across the world that *needs* to acquire the expertise in/of this manual. This manual is designed and designated for both the candidates that are/will primarily not be required to manipulate fractures under anaesthesia and also those that require to, first, manipulate the fracture under anaesthesia to an acceptable anatomical orientation then apply the appropriate POP cast. For clarity's sake the following are the target groups:

1. Students:

    a. Plaster Technicians | Technologists

    b. Nurses

    c. Clinical officers | Clinical assistants | Medical assistants

    d. Physiotherapists/Physiotherapy technologists

    e. Medical students (depending on the period and scheme of study)

        i. Clinical years of study

        ii. Post graduate students in General Surgery and Orthopaedic Surgery

2. Plaster Technicians |Technologists

3. Qualified Nurses – Enrolled Nurses| State Registered Nurses

4. Physiotherapists | Physiotherapy Technologists

5. Clinical officers | Orthopaedic clinical officers

6. Lecturers

    a. Nursing Schools

    b. Post basic nursing schools

    c. Theatre Nursing Schools

    d. Clinical officers | paramedics colleges

    e. Medical schools | Postgraduate medical schools

7. Medical officers

8. General Surgeons

9. Orthopaedic Surgeons

10. Others

Materials [Recipe] for POP application

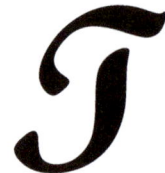The following are the materials needed to easily, effectively and efficiently apply a Plaster of Paris:

1. Plaster of Paris Bandages – various sizes depending on (appropriateness to the)

    a. Patient's age and built

    b. Site of injury

2. Under-cast material

    a. Stockinet (not absolutely necessary)

    b. Cotton wool or Orthopaedic wool

3. Skin lotion (not absolutely necessary)

4. Bucket / Container

5. Kettle or urn

6. Water

7. Pair of POP scissors

8. Surgical blades

9. Incontinent sheet and/or Plaster mat (to protect the patient, linen and the floor)

10. Disposable gloves (may not be necessary – without the gloves, handling of POP with bear hands makes the person applying the cast to do it well and re-live their childhood of playing with plasticine clay!)

11. Plaster or POP room / Plaster OPD/ theatre POP room (Not absolutely necessary) can be done anywhere including the ward

12. Chairs or examination couch

13. Linen / Pillow (may not be necessary)

14. Working surface or trolley or POP table

15. Apron (to protect the technician and the assistant)

16. The injured patient

Mat POP bandage Orthopaedic wool Electric cutter Spreader Manual Shear

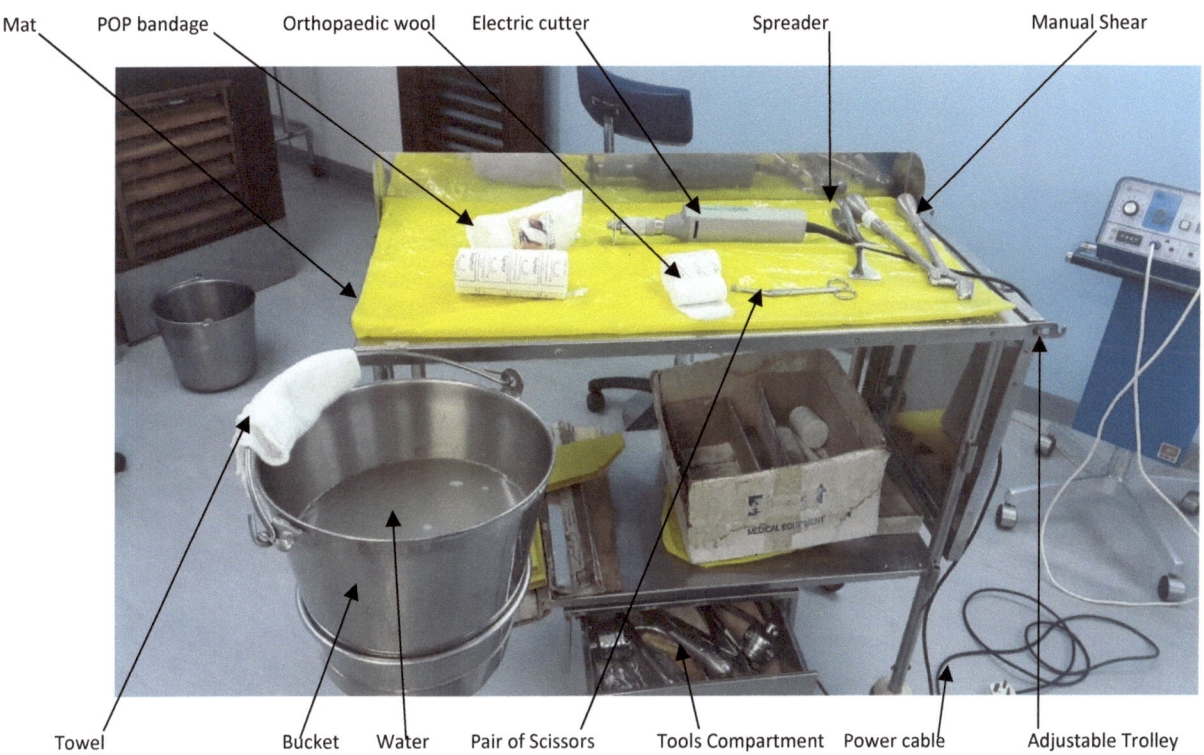

Towel Bucket Water Pair of Scissors Tools Compartment Power cable Adjustable Trolley

"Utensils and ingredients"

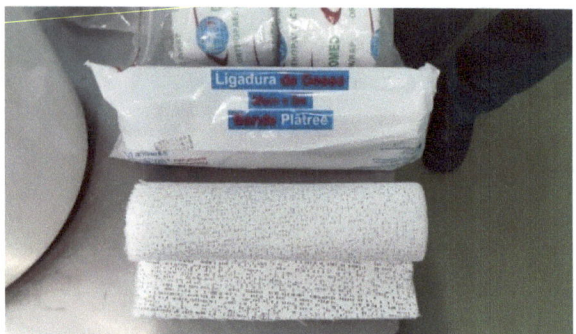

Picture 1: Size 20cm (largest sized POP bandage)

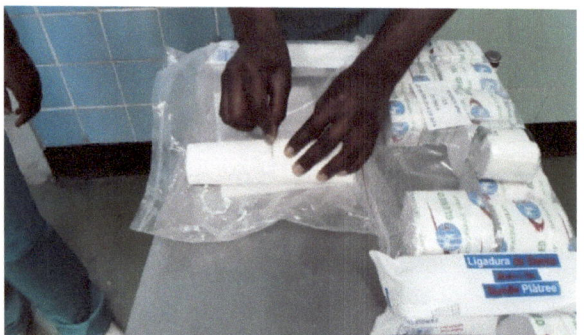

Picture 2: Large POP bandage being cut to "size"

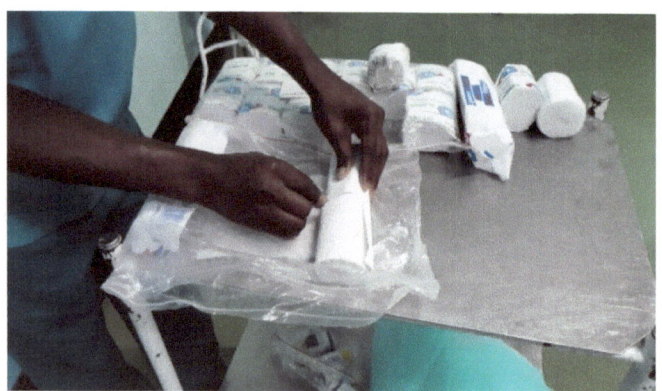

Picture 3: Cutting POP bandage to "size" with a surgical blade to 2x10cms

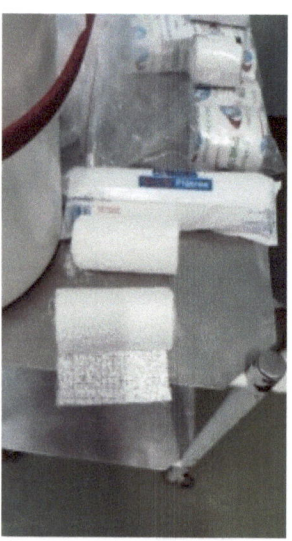

Picture 4: POP bandage cut into 2x10cms

he POP application can be done at/in any place or anywhere. This can be done at a health post (center), in the emergence room, outpatient department, the war, Intensive Care Unit, in the hospital theatre or indeed outside any health/medical infrastructure; e.g. by the road side.

It is however important that a designated place for such a procedure is established at every institution. It is important to do this because the staff will be aware / know where the procedure normally takes place. The situation however can/should dictate where the plaster application will take place on condition that the materials for applying the cast are available and the place is safe for the procedure to be done.

Before one starts or embarks on applying the POP it imperative and important that a thorough preparation for the procedure is done. This is as regards the materials, anticipated POP setting time as well as other factors.

Generally speaking the following must be considered before one starts to apply the POP:

1. Water temperature *(ideal temperature is 22°-25°C—use your elbow to ascertain how warm/"hot" the water is. If your water "burns" the elbow, the water is too "hot"; add more cold water to make it lukewarm(Pictures 11 & 12 below)*

2. Estimated number and size of POP bandages to be used (see "Materials" above)

3. Unwrap / uncover the Plaster of Paris beforehand *(trying to unwrap the POP from its plastic coverings with the hands covered in wet plaster can be difficult unless you have an assistant with dry hands to do it for you)*

4. Placement of POP bandages in relation to the water bucket and the patient's position *(never put or keep your unused exposed bunch of POP bandages between your bucket of water and the working area {limb or the patient}. As you carry a soaked POP bandage from the bucket to the working area, water will drip from the wet POP and hands and will therefore soak bandages on the bunch of exposed and unused POP)— see Figure 1 & 2 below*

5. Comfort of patient, "plaster technician" and assistant: Always make sure that the patient is in a comfortable position as well as the people that are applying the POP.

6. It is advisable that if there are two people applying the cast on a patient, the one who is knowledgeable in the technique must hold the limb and give directions/instructions to the less knowledgeable (who will physically apply the POP) and NOT vice versa.

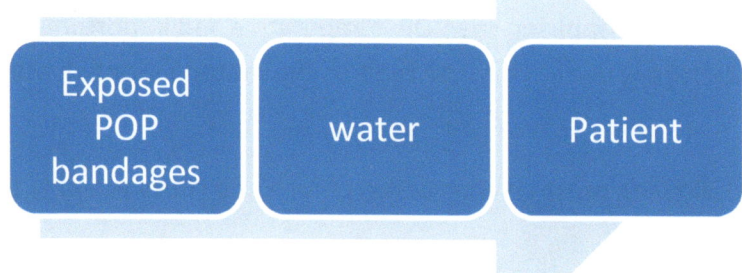

Figure 1: Correct sequence and arrangement of materials (for use) and patient

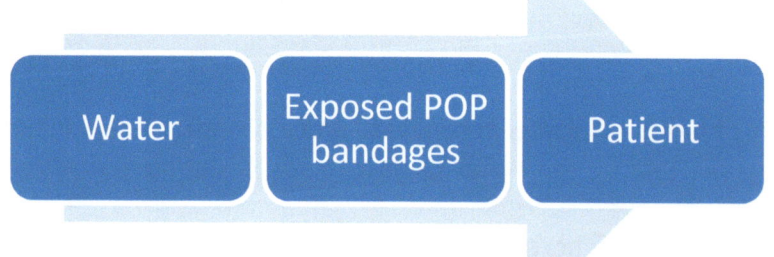

Figure 2: Wrong sequence and arrangement of materials (for use) and patient

Water

Volume of water for use in POP application:

Water for use in the Plaster of Paris application must be adequate enough within the bucket for ease soaking of POP bandages as shown below.

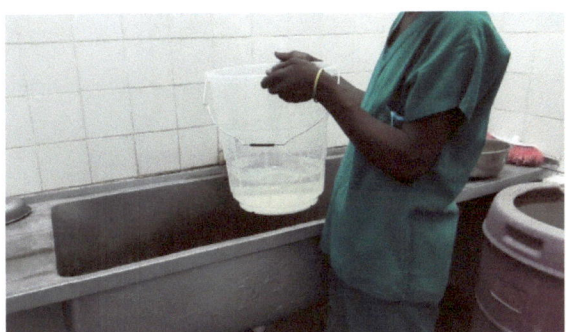

Picture 5: Water is **not adequate** for POP soaking especially the large size

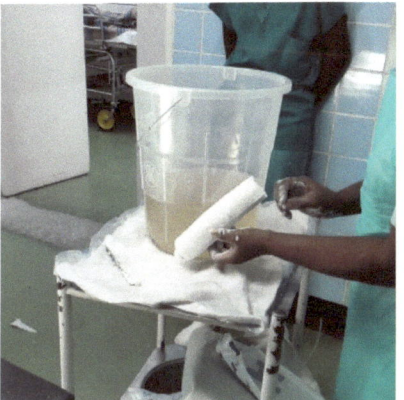

Picture 6: Inadequate water for soaking a 20cm POP

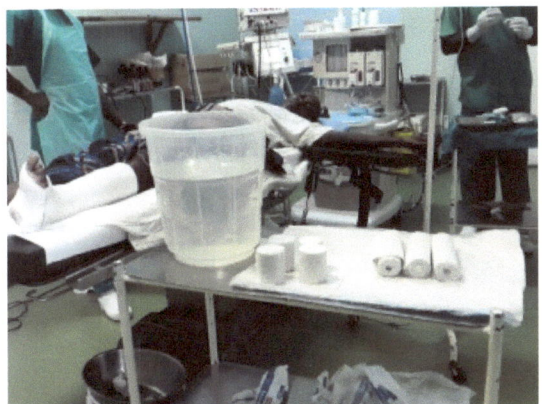

Picture 7: Adequate water in the bucket

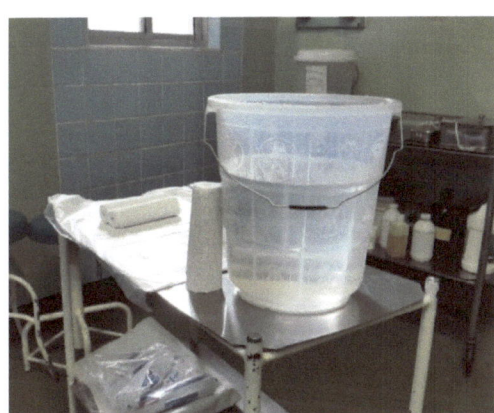

Picture 8: Adequate water for large sized POP (20cm POP)

Mixing of Hot and Cold water:

*D*o not add hot water to the cold water in the bucket; but rather the cold water to the hot water. Hot water is "lighter" than cold water. If hot water is poured onto the cold water, the hot water will "float" over the cold water and this will be dangerous to the one who will dip one's hand into the water as they attempt to soak the POP bandage.

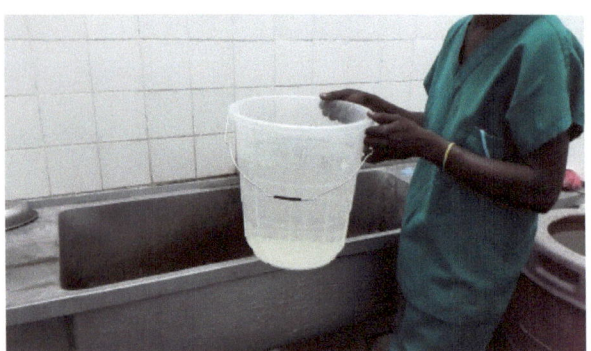

Picture 9: Correct: Cold water to the hot water that is already in the bucket

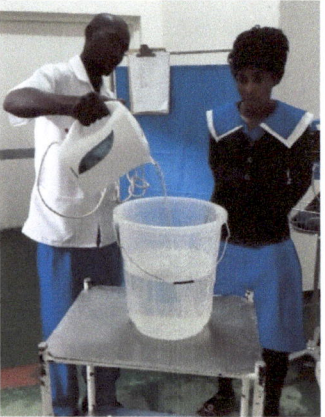

Picture 10: Incorrect: Hot to cold water

Note that cold water is heavier than hot water and will therefore mix easily. If you add hot water to cold water, the hot water will "float" on the cold water and whoever is about to soak the POP in the water may run a risk of burning oneself – be safe!

Water temperature:

The ideal temperature of water for POP application is lukewarm. The technician must dip his/her elbow into the water to feel for the temperature. If it "burns" the elbow, it is too hot for POP application. If, however, it is comfortable on the elbow, then the water temperature is right.

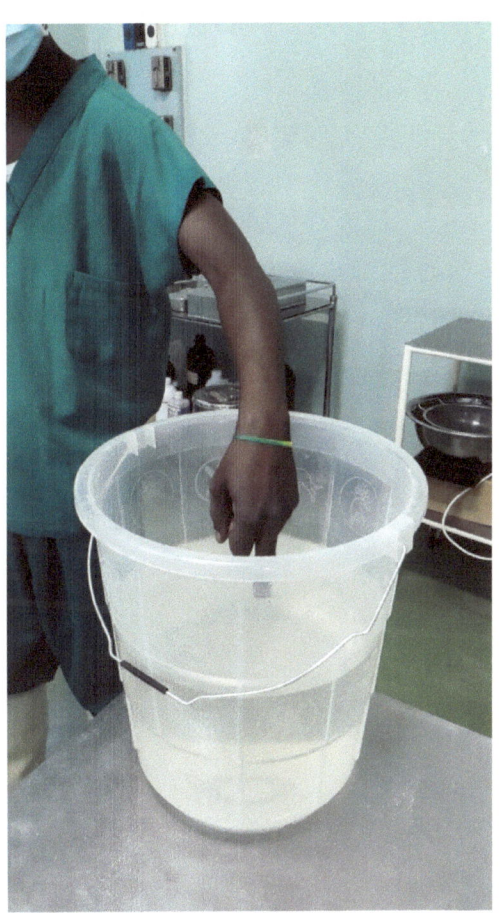

Picture 11: Incorrect - Checking the water temperature

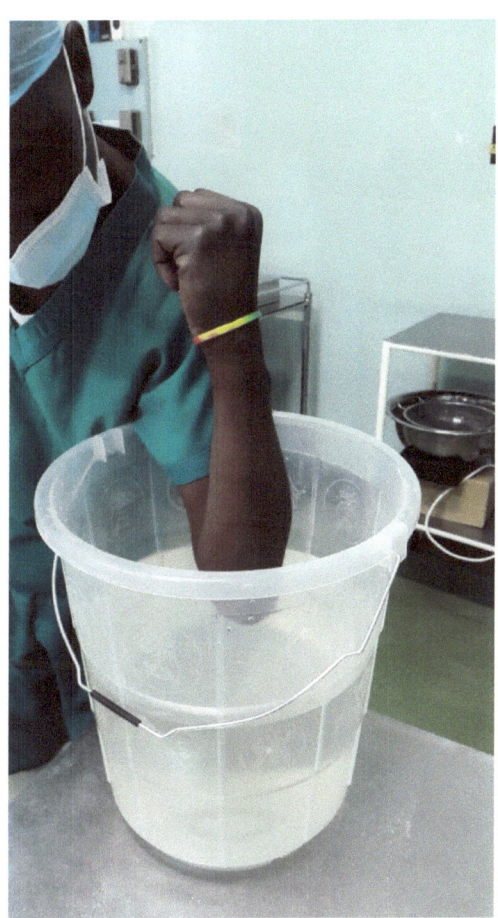

Picture 12: Correct way of checking water temperature

Note: High temperature water reduces the working time with POP (POP will set faster and quickly) and vice versa

Tip (end) of POP plaster:

dentify the end or "tongue" of the POP bandage before it is placed in the bucket of water. It is therefore important to hold the POP with both hands; one hand on the end and the other hand on the whole roll. If you don't do this and soak the whole plaster in the water; it becomes difficult to identify the end of the wet bandage and may result in the POP drying in your hands while trying so hard to locate the plaster bandage end resulting in spoiling the plaster and wastage!

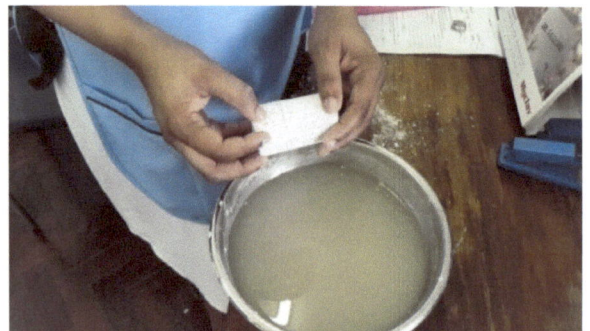

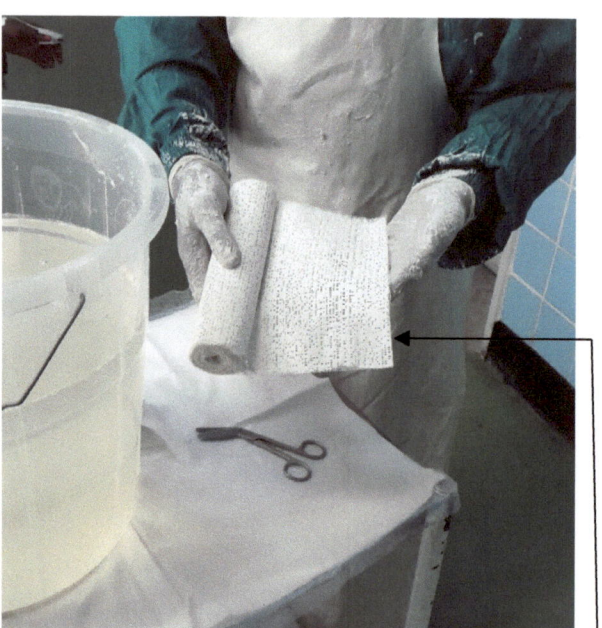

Picture 13: Incorrect; No end identified before soaking it.

Picture 14: Correct way; identify one end   (end of POP)

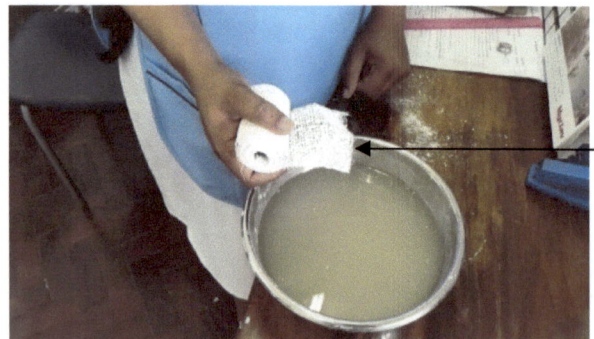

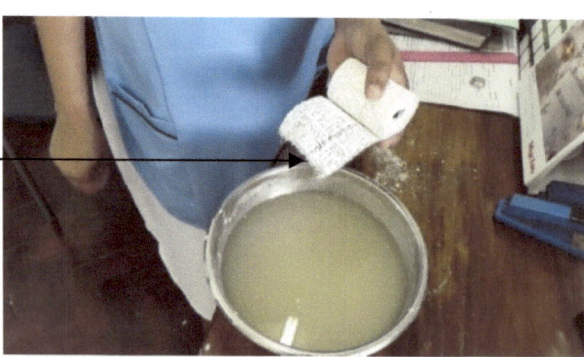

Picture 15A: (Right handed) Correct way before soaking POP   (Pop Ends) **Picture 15B:** Left handed-Correct way: Holding POP just before soaking

Soaking of plaster:

D o not squeeze the bandage as it is being immersed in water as the core of the bandage may not get wet completely, but rather hold it lightly and gently to allow the water to easily permeate and soak deep into the core of the plaster bandage. During the process of immersing or soaking of POP in water, wait for all the air bubbles to stop coming out of the plaster. Once this happens, it is an indication that the POP is completely soaked to the core – *see Picture 16A below*

As you recover/remove the wet POP plaster from the water, ease the water off it gently, on either ends, without literally "squeezing" the POP "dry" as in doing so, much of the plaster will be squeezed off the bandage into the bucket of water (wastage). And secondly, excessive "squeezing" of the POP will allow for reduced working time on that particular over-squeezed "dry-wet" POP bandage and as such the cast might set before the required time (even before molding the cast properly onto the limb) and render the POP cast ineffective and useless – *see Pictures 16C-D below*

With experience, however, one may know when to "squeeze" the wet POP "dry" or otherwise. Therefore, learn the correct method first!

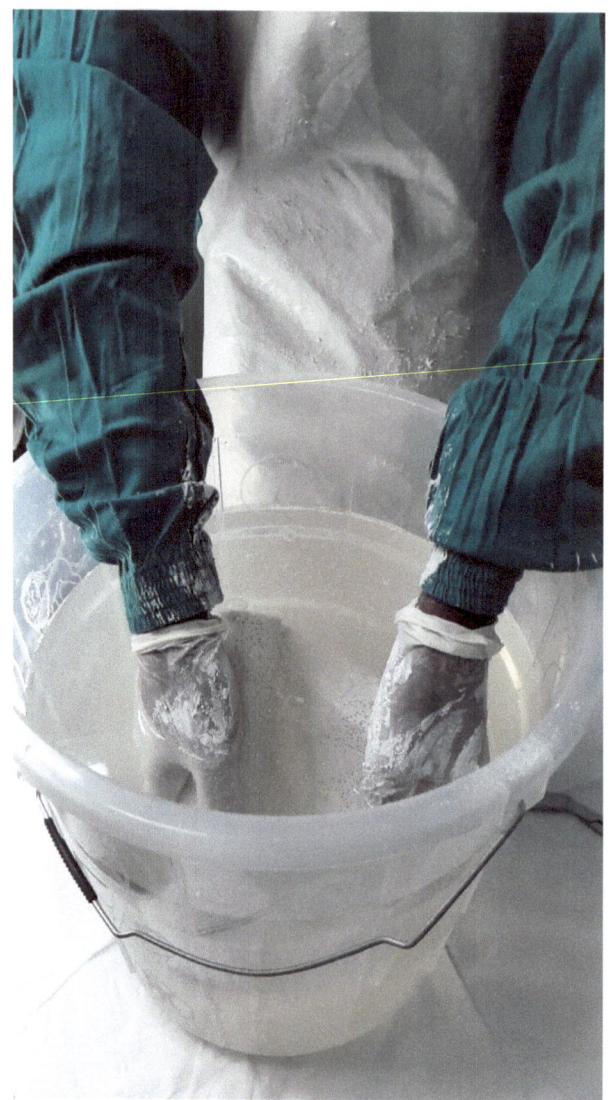

Picture 16A: Completely soaked POP without any emerging air bubbles

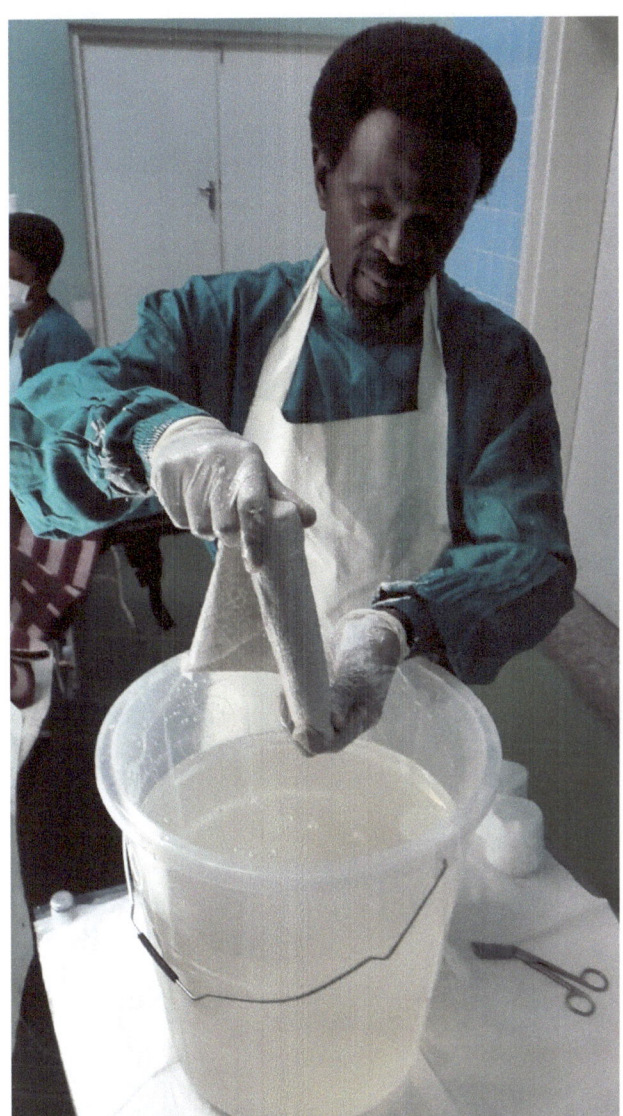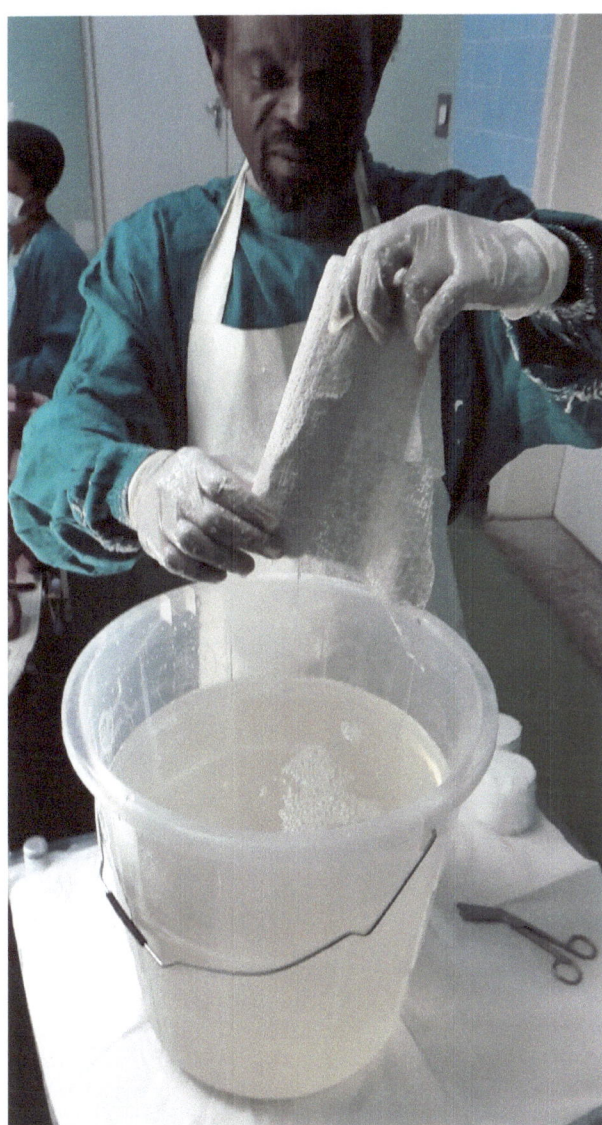

Pictures 16C-D: Gentle easing of water off the soaked POP on either side; with the end clearly identified

Note: Wait for all the water bubbles to stop coming from the immersed POP bandage; this is a sign that the bandage is completely soaked to the core

While it is important to make the patient comfortable before and during the POP application; it must be noted that the limb must be placed in a *functional position* before applying the under-cast, i.e. stockinet, wool or Orthopaedic wool and ultimately the POP. This is important because bending or in deed flexing the joint after the undercast is applied will create *pressure points! These may complicate into decubitus ulcers and infection.* The undercast must therefore be applied in a functional position on and over the joints–*(See Pictures 17 & 18 below)*

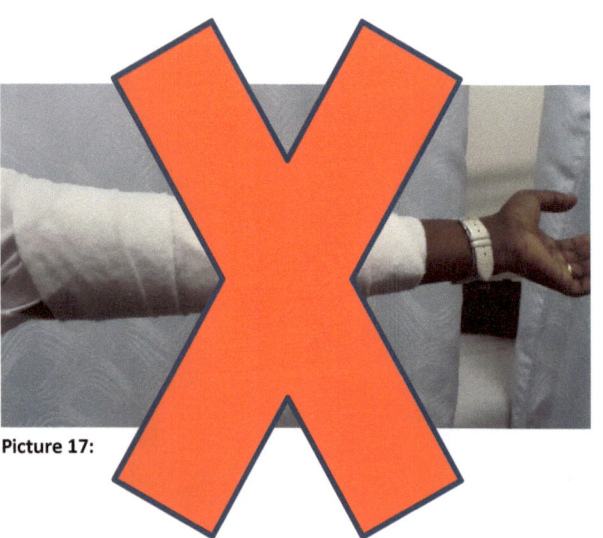

Picture 17:

Pressure point created▢

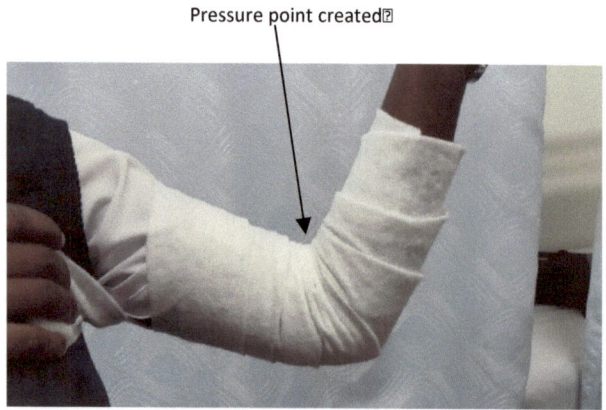

Pictures 18: Elbow flexed – Under cast is kinking (creating pressure point)

To avoid the above situation, the Orthopaedic wool must be applied in a figure of 8 maneuvers over the joints (*see picture 19 & 20 below*).

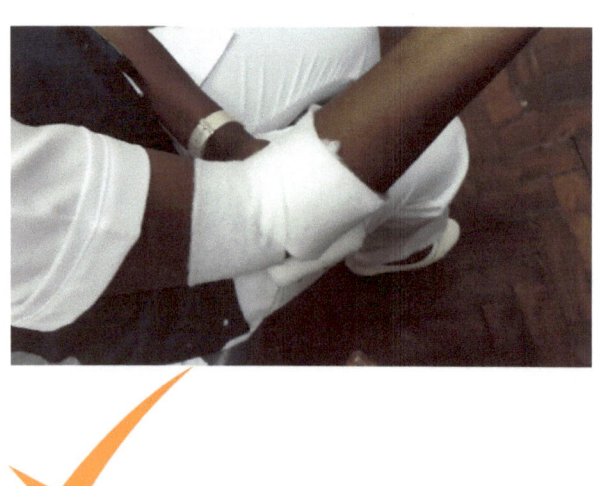

Picture 19: Figure of 8 – Side/Oblique view

Wool applied on an already positioned elbow without wrinkles

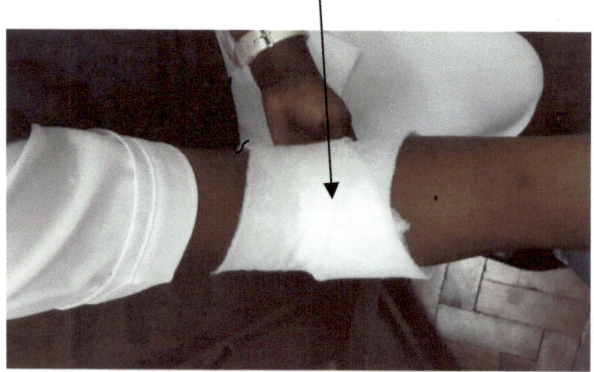

Picture 20: Figure of 8: Front view with elbow flexed – No kinking of wool

Furthermore, all bone prominences must be well padded with Orthopaedic wool to also avoid pressure point effects in these areas and avoid the development of complications (such as decubitus ulcers (pressure soles)).

The areas with bony prominences are around:

1. Wrist joint (head of the ulna)

2. Elbow joint area (medial, lateral and posterior)

3. Ankle joint area (medial, lateral malleoli and the heel) and

4. The knee joint area (anterior (patella), medial and lateral).

Note: Over application of Orthopaedic wool or the undercast wool, however, may render the POP loose and ineffective

The indications and / or contraindications will now be discussed generally. But specific indications and contraindications will again be discussed in specific areas or injuries. The indications, however, of what kind of POP application will vary depending on the following:

a) The severity of injury (personality of injury)

    a. Minor or major trauma

        i. Single or

        ii. Multiple bone involvement (in a limb e.g. the forearm or leg)

    b. Close or open fractures

b) Time of presentation - Early presentation / Late presentation

c) Combination of a) and b) above.

It must be noted here that most fractures that are not displaced are low energy injuries. These however may also present with some degree of oedema (swelling). It is therefore important to recognize this physiological response to trauma as we embark on managing either the soft or hard tissue injuries in these patients.

I f a patient presents to the health facility early enough with a soft or hard tissue injury that require some form of splintage, *do not primarily apply a circular splint!* And in this case an appropriate slab will be indicated. The slab will take its name from the position where it is applied in relation to the anatomical orientation. A slab applied behind the forearm, for example, will be called a back slab. If applied to the front or the lateral sides, it will be called a front / anterior slab and lateral / side slab, respectively; and so on.

The use of a slab is therefore indicated in situations where further swelling of the limb is anticipated. It is used to avert potential complications and is also used as a form of "analgesia" (pain relief).

Some of the anticipated complications in trauma are:

1. Displacement of the fracture

    a. Angulations (anterior, posterior, medial, lateral and other combinations)

    b. Rotation

    c. Overlapping of fracture segments (Telescoping)

    d. Distraction (gap at the fracture site)

    e. Mal-union and Non-union

2. A close fracture complicating into an open fracture

3. Further soft tissue injury if there is a fracture – especially to the neuro-vascular structures

4. Ischaemia of the muscles in the limb or appendage

5. Aggravating symptoms especially and in particular pain

6. Compartment syndrome

7. Amputation of the appendage

Note: Do not apply a circular cast on an acutely injured limb; rather apply an appropriate slab as the primary mode of splintage. This is to avoid compartment syndrome

Table of varied splints or slabs:

Injury	Type of Slab

A Fractured radius or ulna (Single bone)
    a. Distal
    b. Mid shaft
	Below elbow back slab

B Fracture radius and ulna
    a. Distal
    b. Mid shaft
    c. Proximal   - including head of radius
	Above elbow back slab

C Elbow dislocation	Above Elbow back slab
D Humerus Supracondylar fractures (Children)	Above elbow back slab
E Ankle sprain	Below knee back slab +/- U slab
F Tarsal fractures	Below knee back slab +/- U slab
G Metatarsal fractures	Below knee back slab+/- U slab
H Ankle and Pott's fractures	Below Knee back slab +/- U slab
I Tibia or Fibula Fracture	Below Knee back slab
J High Tibia or Fibula fracture	Above knee back slab
K Knee ligamentous injuries	Above Knee back slab
L Fracture Patella (knee cap)	Above knee back slab
M Knee Dislocation (emergence) (after early re-location)	Above Knee back slab
N Distal Femoral Fracture	High above knee back slab

Table 1...

Note1: Other complicated fractures will not be discussed here.

Note2: That a slab and limb elevation are the first lines or choice of treatment in a freshly injured limb (fracture)

Circular casts or POPs will be applied on a limb or on patients that present to the health facility 48 hours or more after the injury and where there is no danger of further limb swelling. Clinical judgment, however, must prevail and be employed on deciding which patient amongst these will require an initial slab splint, for a short period (approximately 48 hours) before a circular cast is applied.

A circular cast is applied as a definitive splint following the primary splintage with a slab. This however may be applied primarily if and when the danger of further limb swelling is eliminated; for example in patients that arrive to the health facility with days of no swelling. Sound, judicious and timely clinical judgment, however, must guide who, and when a circular cast should be applied.

Note that sound clinical assessment and judgment must take precedence before any form of splint is applied

How to apply a slab (Technique)

Materials

1. POP bandages or sheets (layers)

2. Crepe or cotton bandage

3. Under-cast material

   a. Stockinet (not absolutely necessary)

   b. Cotton wool or Orthopaedic wool bandage

4. Skin lotion (not absolutely necessary)

5. Bucket / Container

6. Kettle or urn

7. Water

8. A pair of POP scissors

9. Surgical blades

10. Disposable glove (may not be necessary)

11. Incontinent sheet and / or Plaster mat (to protect the patient, linen and the floor)

12. Plaster or POP room / Plaster OPD room / theatre POP room (Not absolutely necessary) can be done anywhere including the ward

13. Chairs or examination couch

14. Linen / Pillow (may not be necessary)

15. Working surface or trolley

16. Aprons (to protect the technician and the assistant)

17. The injured patient

Technique (General)

The following are general comments. A slab takes/derives its name from the anatomical position where it is applied on the limb. If, for instance, the slab is applied on the posterior (back) aspect of the forearm, it will be called a below elbow back-slab; if on the volar aspect of the forearm, it will be called a volar-slab or anterior or indeed front below elbow slab. If the slab is applied on the lateral aspect or side of the forearm, it will appropriately be called a side or lateral below elbow slab.

Preparation

Prepare all the materials you plan to use before you embark on the exercise.

  a. *Estimate the number of POP bandages that will be used*
  b. *Remove the POP bandages from their plastic coverings*
  c. *Keep the POP away from water (see Figure 1 above)*
  d. *Make sure the water temperature is ideal*
      i. *Hot water shortens the working time while colder water prolongs the working time*
      ii. *"Dry" wet POP shortens the working time, while wetter POP prolongs working time*
  e. *Take measurements from the uninjured corresponding side of the patient (limb)*
  f. *Measure the lengths and thickness of slabs that will be used for a particular procedure beforehand*
  g. *Position the limb and patient appropriately when ready to go!*

Actual Process

The preliminary requirements (as mentioned above) must be observed and followed.

1. The patient is positioned appropriately

2. The site of the slab is identified

3. The length of the slab is measured on the uninjured side using either the Orthopaedic wool or indeed the POP bandage (to avoid causing further pain to the patient if the measurements were done on the injured side). This, however, must be done at a similar site to the injured side while the limb is *positioned in a functional position.*

4. The POP bandage is then measured to the same length and width of the Orthopaedic wool that has been measured and cut according to (3) above. The minimum number of layers of a slab is 9 to 12 layers in children. This however will vary according the age, size and built of a patient.

5. The required number of layers are then soaked (as a thick layer) in water. The POP "thick sheet" is then held in one hand over the bucket or dish of water (see pictures below). The

excess water is gently eased off the edges of this "thick sheet" of POP between the index and long fingers; starting from the top downwards to drain excess water into the bucket.

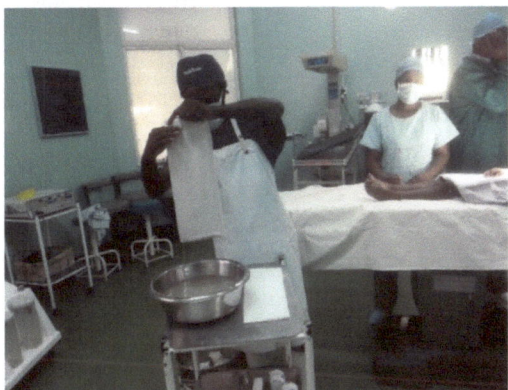 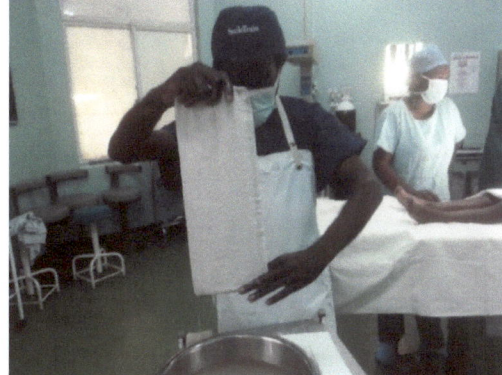

Picture 21A: Gentle easing off the water into the dish (one edge) **Picture 21B:** Easing off the water into the dish (on the other edge of the slab)

6. The thick layer of POP is then laid over the pre-determined layer of Orthopaedic wool (step (3) above); and smoothened out (*avoiding wrinkles* as they are potential pressure points)

7. This is quickly lifted off the working surface (Trolley) and applied onto the desired fracture site. The length and type of the slab will be according to type of injury as indicated in *Table 1 above*.

8. The assistant(s) will hold the slab in position while the "technician" will then apply a roll of either dry crepe/cotton bandage to secure the slab against the fractured appendage/limb. If it is the upper limb involved the maneuver is started around the wrist and worked distally through the first web space; in a similar manner as what is done when applying a wet circular POP. Note that the crepe bandage must be guided through the first web space without it going distal and beyond the level of the distal palmar crease.

9. Once finished applying the crepe or cotton bandage, the end of the bandage is secured with either a wet strip of POP or an Elastoplast / strapping as the case may be.

10. The limb is further and continued held in a functional position while molding the wet slab to the contours of the limb until the slab dries up or sets dry.

11. An arm-sling or collar and cuff is a then applied, if it is on the upper limb. The hand of the affected upper limb (in the slab) must be elevated and rested at the level of the heart. If it is on the lower limb, the foot end of the bed is elevated so that the head end is tilted downwards. The elevation helps to reduce the swelling quickly and give room for an early circular cast to be applied as the subsequent and definitive treatment. The elevated leg/foot must be above the level of the heart.

12. The patient is shown the exercises to perform while the slab is in place. In the upper limbs the patient should be able to flex and extend the fingers freely; and the same for the toes.

13. The patient is examined for any undue tenderness (pain) on passive extension of either the fingers or the toes – *to rule out the impending compartment syndrome!*

14. A patient may be discharged home on a mild analgesia and given instructions of how to look after the slab; for example, not to soak it in water; avoid sitting close to the fire, to come back to the hospital if the pain is getting worse than before the discharge or if the slab becomes very loose that it about to easily fall off the limb.

15. A review appointment date, within 48 to 72 hours, is given to the patient for removal of the slab and replacing it with a circular cast.

Pictures of the hand and foot showing the landmarks where the POP should end

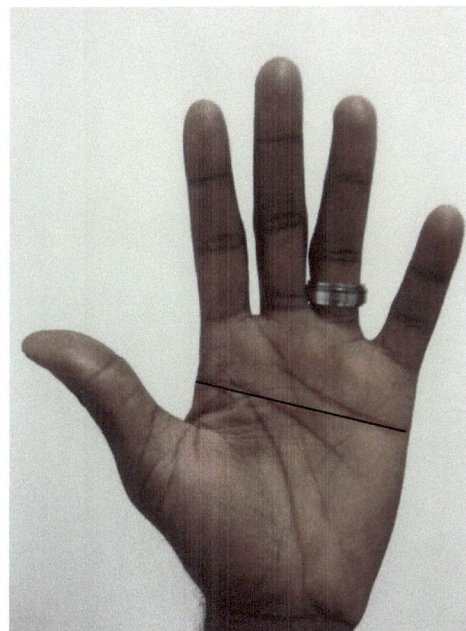

Picture 22A: Landmarks: Distal Palmar crease (hand)

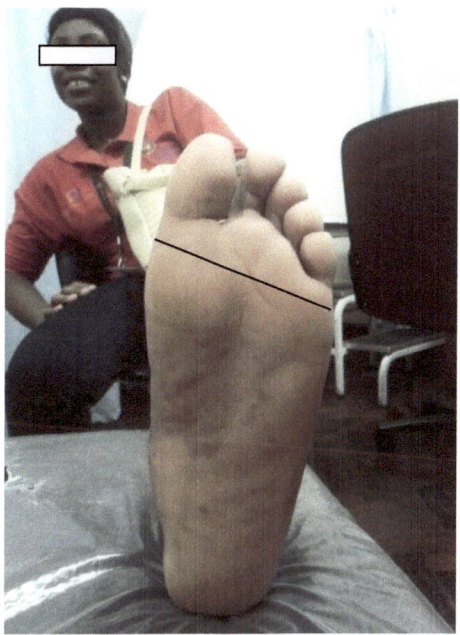

Picture 22B: Distal metatarsal heads (Foot)

Note that the POP must not cross the landmarks indicated above to allow for ease and effective flexion of the fingers (metacarpo-phalangeal joints) and toes (metatarsophalangeal joints) respectively while the limb is within the cast – mobilization!

Upper Limb

Actual Handling and application [Technique – step by step]

Below Elbow back-slab (Forearm)

Materials

1. Appropriate POP bandages or sheets (layers)

2. Crepe or cotton bandage

3. Under-cast material

   a. Stockinet (not absolutely necessary)

   b. Cotton wool or Orthopaedic wool bandage

4. Skin lotion (not absolutely necessary)

5. Bucket / Container

6. Kettle or urn

7. Water

8. A pair of POP scissors

9. Surgical blades

10. Disposable glove (may not be necessary) – Personal protective equipment (PPE)

11. Incontinent sheet and / or Plaster mat (to protect the patient, linen and the floor) - PPE

12. Plaster or POP room / Plaster OPD room / theatre POP room (Not absolutely necessary) can be done anywhere including the ward

13. Chairs or examination couch

14. Linen / Pillow (may not be necessary)

15. Working surface or trolley

16. Aprons (to protect the technician and the assistant) - PPE

17. The injured patient

The preliminary requirements and indications must be observed and followed. This is one of the commonly applied slabs in the clinics/hospitals, both in children and adults. The following are some of the indications:

a. Mid shaft radial fracture or mid shaft ulna fracture

b. Distal ulna or radius fractures

c. Colles', Smith's or Burton's fractures (distal radius fractures before manipulation under anaesthesia)

d. Wrist sprain

e. Metacarpal bone fractures

Preparation

Prepare all the materials you plan to use before you embark on the exercise.

    a. *Estimate the number of POP bandages that will be used*
    b. *Remove the POP bandages from their plastic coverings*
    c. *Keep the POP away from water (see Figure 1 on pp 20 above)*
    d. *Make sure the water temperature is ideal*
        i. *Hot water shortens the working time while colder water prolongs the working time*
        ii. *"Dry" wet POP shortens the working time, while wetter POP prolongs working time*
    e. *Take measurements from the uninjured corresponding side of the patient (limb)*
    f. *Measure the lengths and thickness of slabs that will be used for a particular procedure beforehand*
    g. *Position the limb and patient appropriately when ready to go!*

Actual Process

1. The patient is positioned appropriately.

    a. The patient can be seated on a chair, with the injured elbow resting on/by the edge of the couch or a table and being supported by the un-injured hand *(see picture 32 below)* or

    b. The patient can lie in a supine position with the arm and elbow of the injured limb resting on a pillow with the injured forearm elevated vertically with or without support of the uninjured hand. The palm of the injured hand must be towards the patient's face, while the technician stands toward the dorsal side of the hand, wrist and forearm; on the same side as the injury.

2. The site of the slab is identified – the back-slab

3. The length of the slab is measured on the uninjured side using either the Orthopaedic wool or indeed the POP bandage (this is to avoid causing further pain to the patient if the measurement was done on the injured side); this "template" must be *positioned in a functional position, with the wrist at approximately 45° in extension.* The measurement must be from the Olecranon or 4 fingers distal to the Olecranon to 2cm from the knuckles.

4. The POP bandage is then measured to the same length and width of the Orthopaedic wool that has been pre-measured and cut according to (3) above. The minimum number of layers of a slab is 9 to 12 layers in children and more in adults. This however will vary according the age, size and built of a patient.

5. The required number of layers are then soaked (as a thick layer) in water. The POP "sheet" is then held in one hand over the bucket of water. The excess water is gently eased off the edges of this longitudinal layer of "sheet" of POP starting from the top downwards to drain excess water off it into the bucket.

6. The thick layer of POP is then laid over the pre-determined layer of Orthopaedic wool (step (3) above); and smoothened out (*avoiding wrinkles* as they are potential pressure points)

7. This is then quickly lifted off the working surface (Trolley) and applied onto the desired fractured limb – on the back or posterior aspect of the forearm. The length of the slab will be according to (3) above.

8. The assistant(s) will hold the slab in position while the "technician" will then apply a roll of either dry crepe/cotton bandage to secure the slab against the fractured forearm. The circular maneuver begins at the wrist with two motions to secure the slab and then towards the hand and through the first web space in a similar manner as what is done when applying a wet circular POP. It is easier to start from the volar wrist, over the radial side and to the dorsal wrist and come round the ulna side back to the front. This motion is repeated and towards the back of the hand. The technician holds the bulk of the crepe/cotton bandage in one hand and gathers the broad crepe or cotton bandage between his/her index finger and the thumb in the other hand through the patient's first web space; just before (proximal to) the distal palmar crease on the volar side. The bandage is then spread out to cover the dorsal (posterior or back of the hand) with the distal edge just 2cm short of the knuckles.

9. The bandage is then applied towards the elbow, until it is securely applied. Once finished applying the crepe or cotton bandage, the end of the bandage is secured with either a wet strip of POP or an Elastoplast/strapping as the case may be.

10. The limb is then held is such a way that it is in a function position while molding the wet slab to the contours of the forearm until the slab dries up or sets dry.

11. An arm-sling or collar & cuff is a then applied to support the forearm around the neck. The hand of the injured forearm (in the slab) must be at the level of the heart. This helps to elevate the limb which in turn helps to quickly reduce the swelling in the forearm and leave room for an early circular cast for a subsequent and definitive treatment.

12. The patient is shown the exercises to perform while the slab is in situ. The patient should be able to flex and extend the fingers freely.

13. The patient is examined for any undue tenderness (pain) on passive extension of the fingers – *to rule out the impending compartment syndrome!*

14. A patient may be discharged home on a mild analgesia and given instructions of how to look after the slab; for example, not to soak it in water; avoid sitting close to the fire, and to report back to the hospital if the pain is getting worse than before the discharge or if the slab becomes very loose that it can easily fall off the forearm.

15. A review appointment date, within 48 to 72 hours, is given to the patient for removal of the slab and replacing it with a circular cast.

Extension Block Splint (Burke Halter)

This is a special double-splint indicated for fractures of the short long bones of the fingers; the proximal and / or middle phalanges. It is applied to a single or multiple proximal or middle phalangeal fractures. Prior to the application of this splint, it is important to make sure that the fingers are in the correct anatomical orientation. The finger nails must all be in the same plane. The injured finger, closed or open, must be splinted next to the adjacent uninjured finger. This is called "buddy-splintage" or "buddy splinting".

When a soldier is wounded on the battle field, the other soldier does not abandon the injured. The injured is carried to safety by his buddy!

The uninjured finger in this case helps to "carry" the injured in the "buddy-splintage" and helps mobilize the injured finger.

To apply this splintage the following materials are required:

Materials

1. Appropriate POP bandages or sheets (layers)

2. Crepe or cotton bandage

3. Under-cast material

    a. Stockinet (not absolutely necessary)

    b. Cotton wool or Orthopaedic wool bandage

4. Skin lotion (not absolutely necessary)

5. Bucket / Container

6. Kettle or urn

7. Water

8. A pair of POP scissors

9. Surgical blades

10. Disposable glove (may not be necessary) – Personal Protective Equipment (PPE)

11. Incontinent sheet and / or Plaster mat (to protect the patient, linen and the floor) – PPE

12. Plaster or POP room / Plaster OPD-room / theatre POP room (Not absolutely necessary) can be done anywhere including the ward

13. Chairs or examination couch

14. Linen / Pillow (may not be necessary)

15. Working surface or trolley

16. Aprons (to protect the technician and the assistant) – PPE

17. The injured patient

Actual application of the Extension Block Splint

Preparation

Prepare all the materials you plan to use before you embark on the exercise.

   a. *Estimate the number of POP bandages that will be used*
   b. *Remove the POP bandages from their plastic coverings*
   c. *Keep the POP away from water (see Figure 1 above)*
   d. *Make sure the water temperature is ideal*
       i. *Hot water shortens the working time while colder water prolongs the working time*
       ii. *"Dry" wet POP shortens the working time, while wetter POP prolongs working time*
   e. *Take measurements from the uninjured corresponding side of the patient (limb)*
   f. *Measure the lengths and thickness of slabs that will be used for a particular procedure beforehand*
   g. *Position the limb and patient appropriately when ready to go!*

Actual Process

1. Measure the length of the front slab using an Orthopaedic wool bandage or indeed the POP bandage, wide enough to cover the front of the forearm; from the distal palmar crease to 2cm short of the cubital fossa (with the wrist in extension (~45°– 60°). Nine to 12 layers of POP are measured to length and set aside.

   a. In a similar manner, measure a layer of Orthopaedic wool bandage from the tip of the fingers to just short of the tip of the Olecranon (on the dorsal aspect of the forearm – back-slab) with the wrist in extension (~45° – 60°) while the carpo-metacarpal joints are at about 90°. Again, set this aside. At this point you will have:

       i. The front single or double layer of Orthopaedic wool for the front forearm

       ii. The front 9-12 un-soaked layers of POP for the front forearm

       iii. The posterior or dorsal single or double layer of Orthopaedic wool bandage for the forearm

       iv. The posterior or dorsal 9-12 un-soaked layers of POP for the forearm

   b. The injured finger is secured in a buddy-splint using a tape or Elastoplast (with a thin layer of gauze between the injured and buddy fingers)

c. Soak the front POP slab layers completely and ease off the excess water into the bucket

d. Apply the wet POP layer onto the Orthopaedic wool bandage. Lift the "Buttered" wet slab with wool and apply it with the Orthopaedic wool bandage against the forearm skin. The assistant holds the slab against the palm ending at the distal palmar crease with the patient's wrist in extension while supporting his elbow on the edge of the couch or trolley (*like in picture 32*). Remember that the patient is in a sitting position with his palm face-ward. The assistant is standing on the right side of the patient (if the right hand is injured) while the technician stands opposite the assistant across the end of the couch.

e. The technician then applies a wet or dry crepe bandage to secure the slab starting from the wrist into the hand and down to the wrist and end up down near the elbow.

f. The technician then molds the slab along the front of the forearm while maintaining the extended wrist. Make sure the front or volar slab sets *before* the posterior or dorsal slab is applied. This allows for a better result.

g. Repeat steps (3) and (4) above for the dorsal slab. Secure the posterior (dorsal) slab with the wrist in extension (45° to 60°) while the metacarpo-phalangeal joints positioned at about 90°.

h. Twenty-four hours later, the crepe bandage is trimmed off the volar aspect of the fingers to expose them so as to allow for early finger mobilization (flexion and extension).

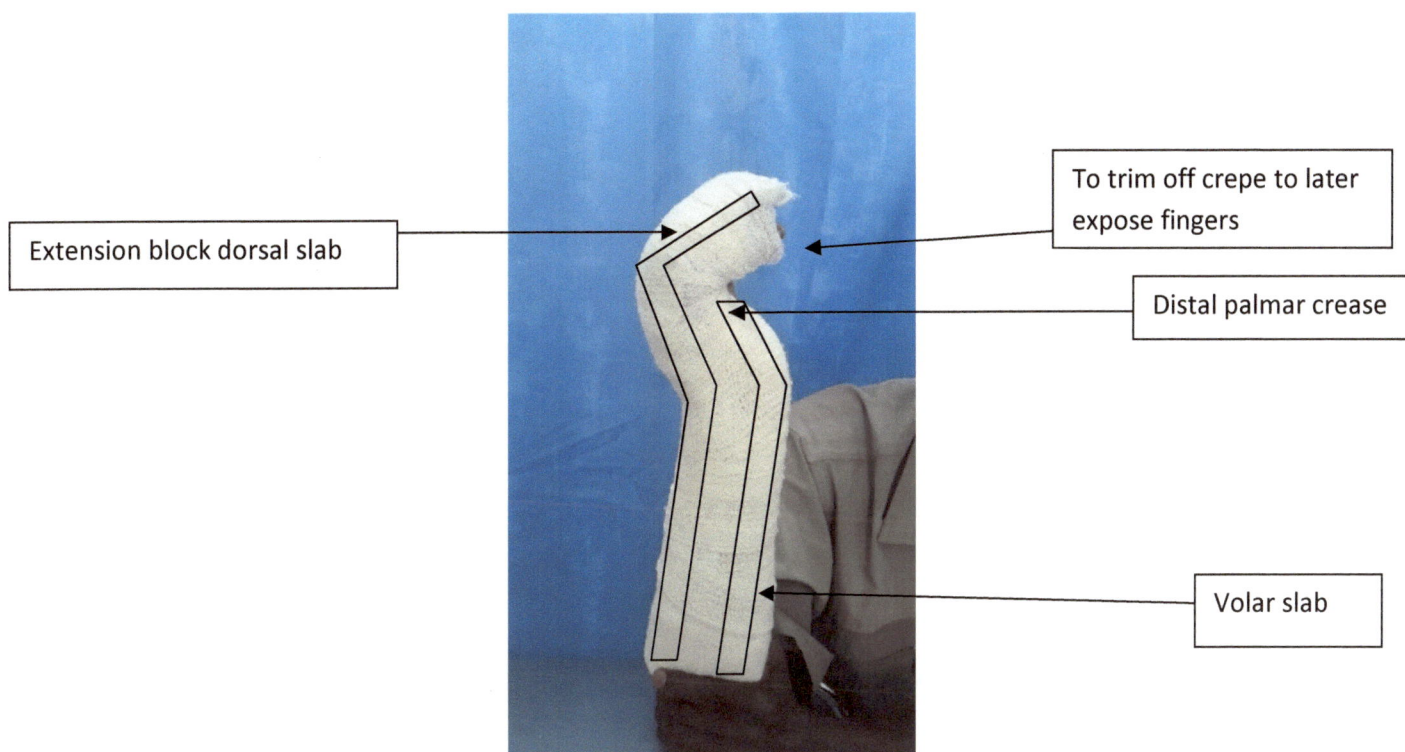

Extension block dorsal slab

To trim off crepe to later expose fingers

Distal palmar crease

Volar slab

Figure 3...

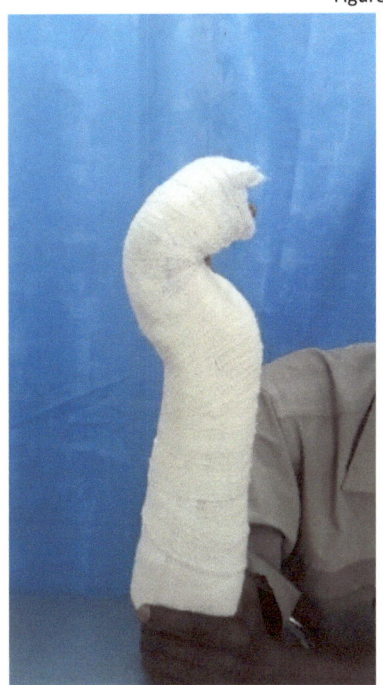

Picture 24: Medial view

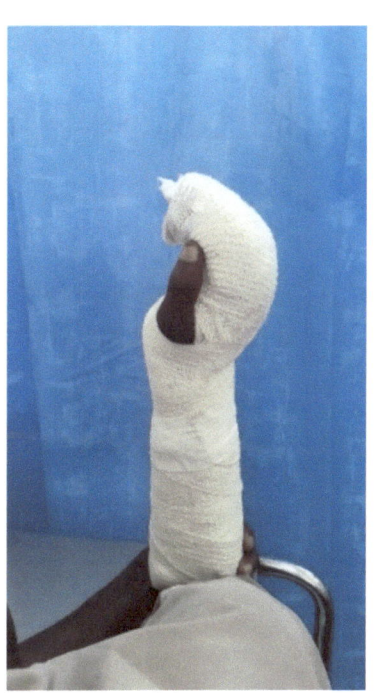

Picture 25: Lateral view

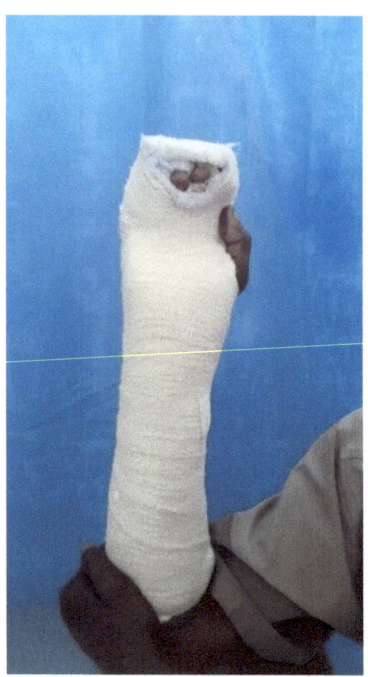

Picture 26: Frontview before cutting off the crepe

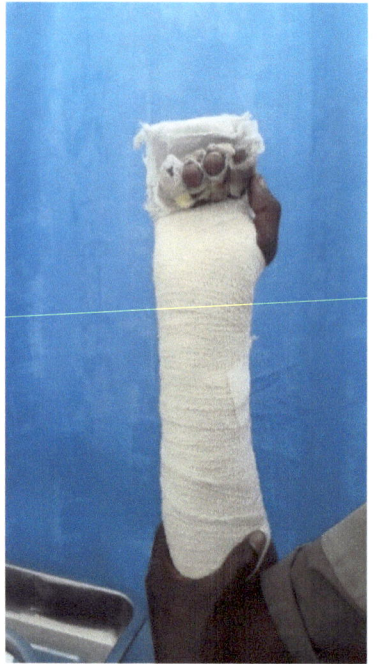

Picture 27: Front view with exposed fingers

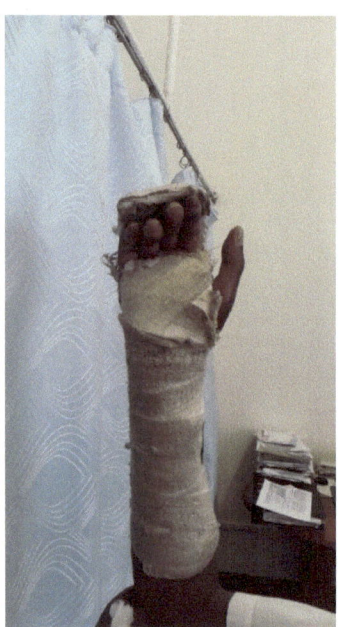

Picture 28A: At four weeks post injury

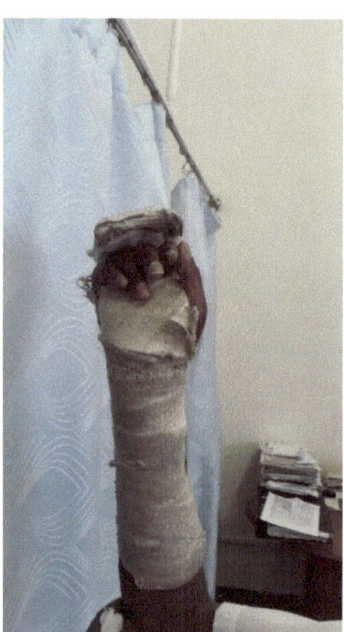

Picture 28B: Finger-flexion at 4 weeks post injury

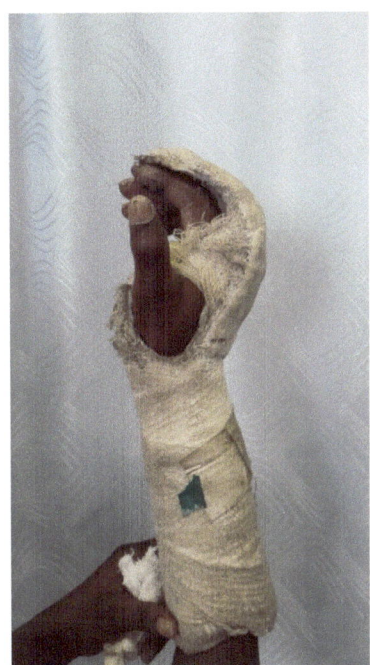

Picture 28C: Fingers in extension (4/52 post injury)

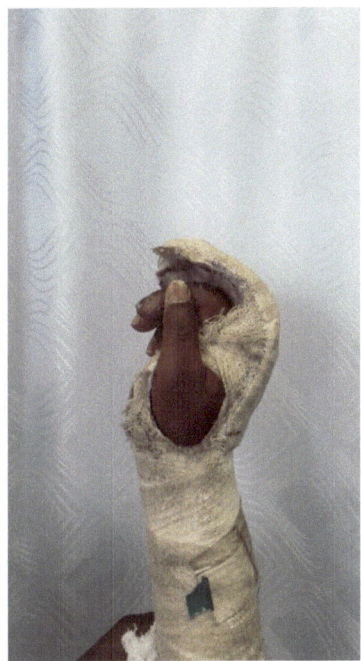

Picture 28D: Flexion – 4 weeks post injury

Direction of unrolling (applying) the POP bandage onto the limb:

Easy unrolling of the wet POP bandage makes the application of the cast easier and simpler. This is illustrated in the following pictures. The Orthopaedic wool, crepe bandage, cotton bandage and indeed the wet Plaster of Paris bandage are easily applied by unrolling them in the direction illustrated below (*Pictures 29C-D*).

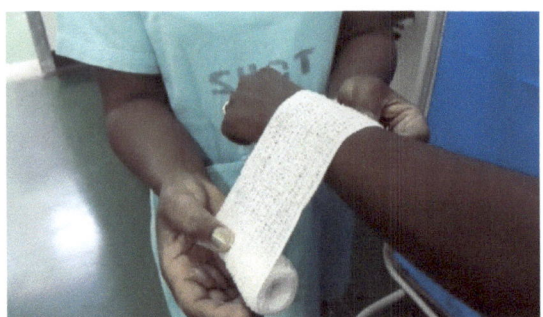 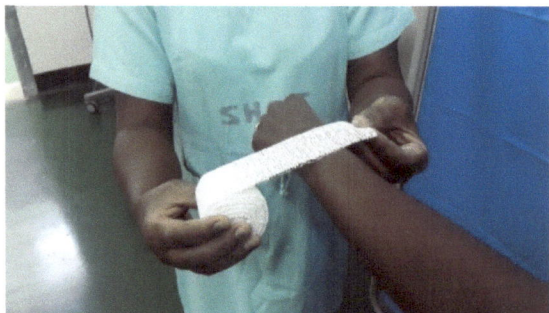

Pictures 29 A-B: Incorrect direction (applying) of unrolling an Orthopaedic wool bandage (not in picture), crepe bandage or Plaster of Paris on the limb

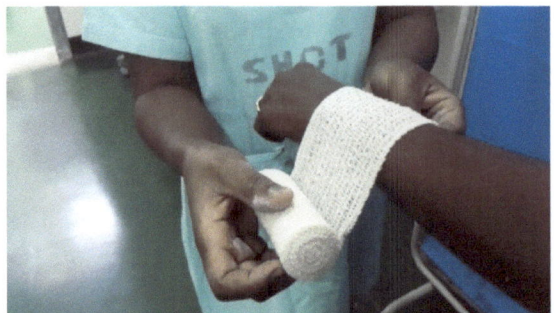 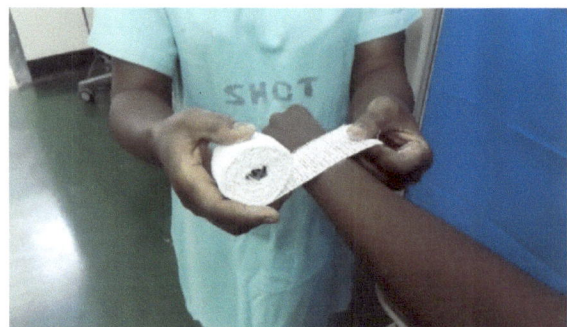

Picture 29C-D: Correct direction (applying) or unrolling an Orthopaedic wool bandage (not in picture), crepe bandage or Plaster of Paris

Note that the crepe bandage must not be pulled tight on a limb; it will otherwise compromised the venous, and if tighter the arterial circulation in a limb

*I*t is advisable to begin applying the POP near the wrist in the upper limb and work your way down to the hand and up towards the elbow. On the lower limb, it is advisable to start from the foot and work your way upwards, proximally.

POP handling (The actual application):

*H*old the "whole" POP bandage roll in one hand and smoothen the area just applied with the other. This helps to push/press the air bubbles trapped under and between the POP layers out and allows the POP "hold" together as one solid layer and avoid the "onion peel effect" with individual layers that results into a poor plaster setting.

The smallest sized POP (5cm) bandage must be held by the edges; between the thumb and the index; or thumb and index and long fingers as illustrated below. This is to avoid the POP bandage ending up forming a "thread" instead of it being spread out in its full width as it is being applied. If the latter happens, it will lead to wastage (discarding the threaded plaster)!

Hold POP between thumb and fingers

Small POP easily form a "Thread"

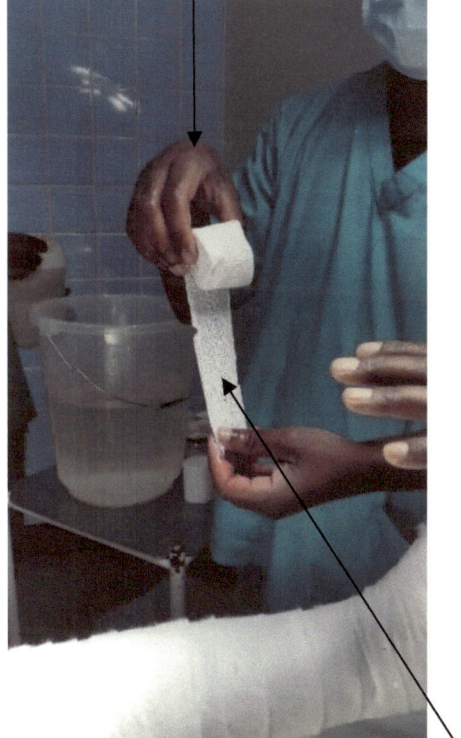

"Broad" POP;

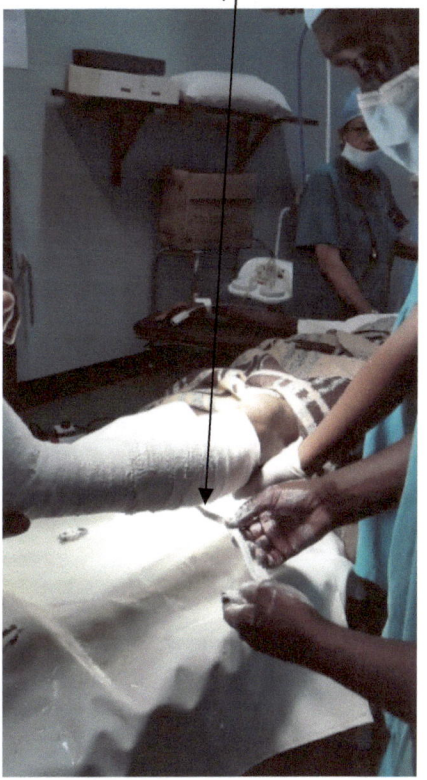

Picture 30A: Holding of the smallest sized POP bandage (5cm width) between index/long fingers and thumb

Picture 30B: When poorly handled it forms a "thread" before applying it on a limb – leading to wastage.

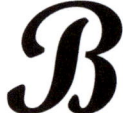egin the application of the next wet POP bandage from where the earlier one ended; this allows achieving an evenly applied and aesthetically looking and acceptable cast.

Immediate Post POP application (Aftermath)

𝒶 chemical reaction takes place when POP gets in contact with water; and heat is emitted. It is important to inform the patient about this experience so that (s)he is aware. And it is therefore important not to use water that is hot (above 22°– 25°C) as this may burn the patient.

At the end of the procedure

𝒥t is important to clean the limb of the patient at the end of the application procedure of the Plaster cast, as the parts of the limb out of the POP cast will be soiled or "stained" in POP. This looks untidy; hence the need to clean the patient. This is usually well received by patients and allows good working rapport to develop between the patient and the medical staff.

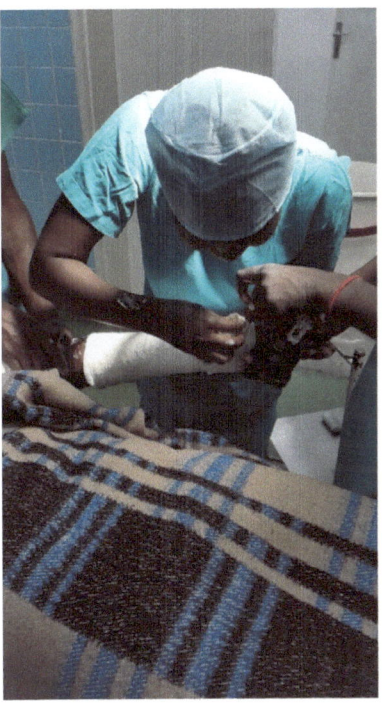

Picture 31 A: Cleaning the patient

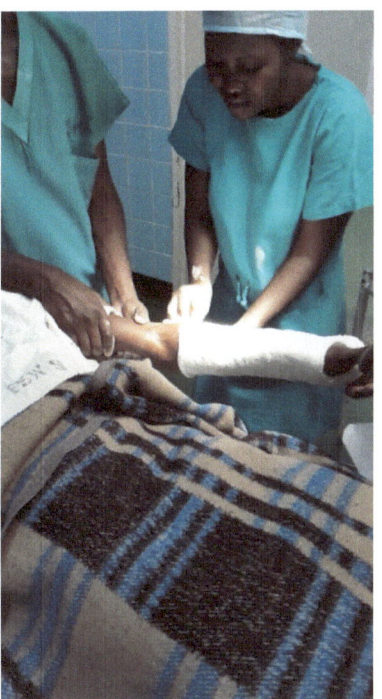

Picture 31 B: Cleaning the proximal end

Circular Cast

Below Elbow Circular Cast or POP

Actual Handling and application [Technique]

Materials

The following are the materials needed to easily and effectively apply a Plaster of Paris:

1. Plaster of Paris Bandages – various sizes depending on (appropriateness to the)

    a. Patient's age and built

    b. Site for application

Note: It is better to stock the largest/biggest size of POP bandage than the smaller size. If small sized POP plaster is needed for use, the larger size can be cut to the appropriate size needed for the job. The best is to have all the sizes available!

2. Under-cast material

    a. Stockinet (not absolutely necessary)

    b. Cotton wool or Orthopaedic wool bandage

3. Skin lotion (not absolutely necessary)

4. Bucket / Container

5. Kettle or urn

6. Water

7. A pair of POP scissors

8. Surgical blades

9. Incontinent sheet and / or Plaster mat (to protect the patient, linen and the floor)

10. Disposable gloves (may not be necessary)

11. Plaster or POP room / Plaster OPD / theatre POP room (Not absolutely necessary) can be done anywhere including the ward

12. Chairs or examination couch

13. Linen / Pillow (may not be necessary)

14. Working surface or trolley

15. Apron (to protect the technician and the assistant)

16. The injured patient

Preparation

Prepare all the materials you plan to use before you embark on the exercise.

a. *Estimate the number of POP bandages that will be used*
b. *Remove the POP bandages from their plastic coverings*
c. *Keep the POP away from water (see Figure 1 above)*
d. *Make sure the water temperature is ideal*
    i. *Hot water shortens the working time while colder water prolongs the working time*
    ii. *"Dry" wet POP shortens the working time, while wetter POP prolongs working time*
e. *Take measurements from the uninjured corresponding side of the patient (limb)*
f. *Measure the lengths and thickness of slabs that will be used for a particular procedure beforehand*
g. *Position the limb and patient appropriately when ready to go!*

Actual Process

1. This plaster is best applied when the patient is seated with the elbow rested on the edge of a table or a couch and the technician in front of the patient. This allows the technician full access to the limb. The plaster can be applied with or without an assistant. If the assistant is not available, the patient can support his/her injured hand with the uninjured hand – with prior education and demonstration; *see picture 32 below.*

2. Apply the stockinet (if not available, it is not really necessary) and under-cast slightly over the intended edge of the final POP with the wrist in a functional position.

3. The landmarks:

    a. The distal palmar crease in the hand and

    b. 2-finger breadth from the cubital fossa at the elbow.

    The above landmarks will allow the patient to freely flex the fingers through the metacarpo-phalangeal joints and the elbow respectively, while in the below elbow POP cast

4. The indication for a below elbow POP have been shown above – both for children and adults.

5. Hold the POP in both hands; one hand holding the whole POP bandage roll, while the other takes the tip or end of the cast as shown in the earlier picture before soaking it. This is important as you will be able to identify the one end of the POP bandage before it is soaked. If the above is not done, one may lose sight of where the end is. As one keeps looking for the end on the wet bandage, the POP may end up drying and later discarded as spoilt. In some hospitals patients are made to buy the POP from outside the hospital. This will therefore be an

unnecessary cost to the patient, especially in economically challenged societies. This may also be an unnecessary cost to the hospital and the ministry of health if the hospital provides the POP.

6. Soak the POP bandage completely. Do not however squeeze the POP into the bucket, but rather just ease off the excess water gently down into the bucket. Then start applying from the wrist area. Go firmly around the wrist twice and proceed distally towards the hand (not beyond the distal palmar crease). As one maneuvers the POP in the first web space (between one's Index finger and the Thumb), one must gather or pinch the POP between your thumb and index finger in one hand while the whole roll of POP bandage will be in another. Do this twice and proceed proximally. The POP must overlap 50% as it is being applied. The air bubbles are express out of the POP as you smoothen the POP with one hand while the roll is in the other hand; and vice versa. This helps the POP to set as "one" and does not exhibit the "onion peel effect".

7. After the ends (proximal and distal) have been secured, the protruding stockinet/under-cast can then be folded back over the edge of the POP. This will prevent the POP from injuring the adjacent skin from the rough POP edges but give the final cast a smooth soft edge and finish (by the cubital fossa and the distal palmar crease).

8. The POP should not be "cylindrical" and if left like this the POP may easily "slide" off the forearm. It is therefore imperative to mold the plaster over the contours of the forearm with slight wrist extension. Between the mid 1/3 of the forearm to the wrist the POP must assume an oval shape while the proximal 1/3 will be more circular (in a cross-section). Note that the distal half of the forearm is flattish.

9. Once the POP sets, the forearm is placed in an arm-sling with its hand held at the level of the heart while the elbow will be flexed.

10. The patient will be given instructions on how to look after the POP e.g.

    a. Don't not soak the POP in water or any liquids

    b. Keep the forearm elevated in the sling

    c. Report back to the hospital if the POP feels too tight and begins to hurt more

    d. Mobilize the joints that are outside and not included in the or under the cast

    e. Avoid exposing the cast to extreme levels of heat, as this may lead to thermal injuries

    f. Avoid poking the under surface of the plaster because of the itchiness that follows. This act may push the under-casting into forming a lump which will be a pressure point within the cast

g. When the POP feels loose, the patient must return to the health facility so that a well-fitting one is re-applied

h. To report back to the health facility whenever in doubt over anything related to the injury and the treatment

11. Discharge patient on pain relieving medication (appropriate analgesia)

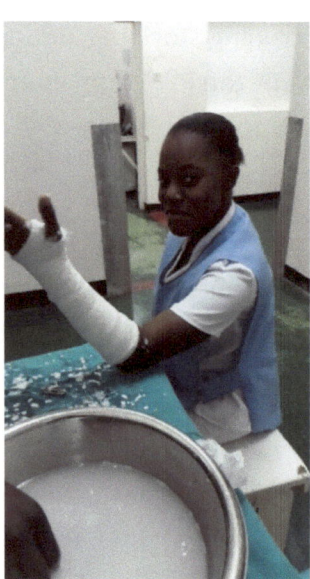

Picture 32: Forearm resting on the edge of the table for ease of application

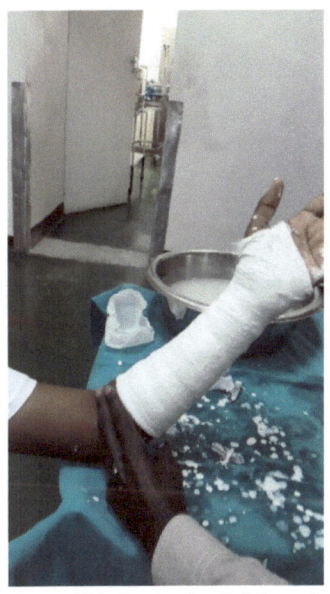

Picture 32A: Proximal end: 2-finger breadth from the cubital fossa

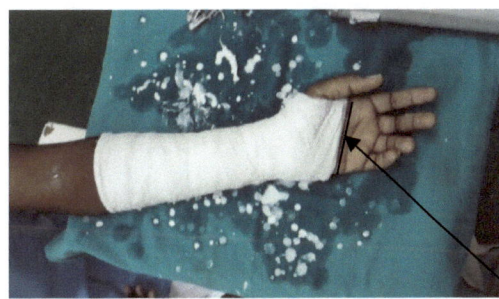

Distal Palmar crease

Picture 32B: Distal end: Along distal palmar crease; Free thumb base

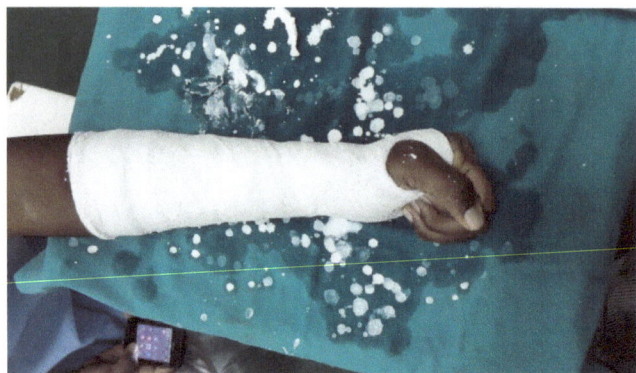

Picture 33A: Able to clench a fist (Top view)

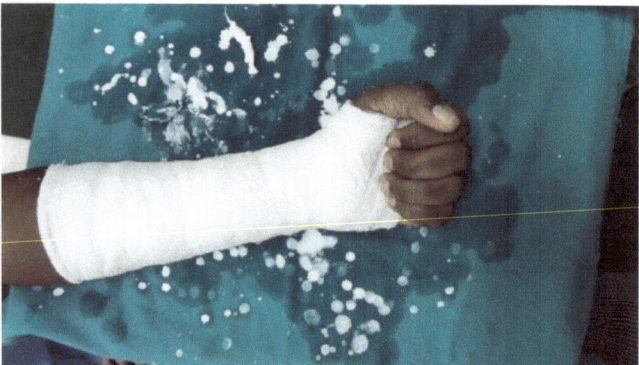

Picture 33B: Able to clench a fist (Front view)

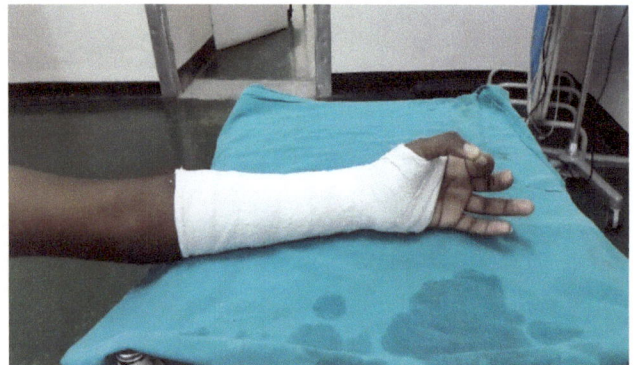

Picture 34A: Apposition of the thumb against the index finger

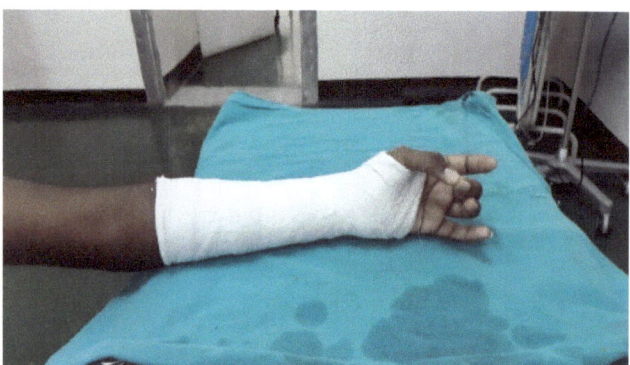

Picture 34B: Apposition of the thumb against the long finger

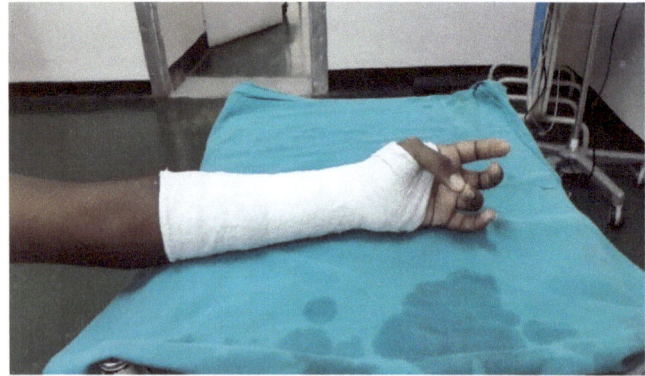

Picture 34C: Apposition of the thumb against the ring finger

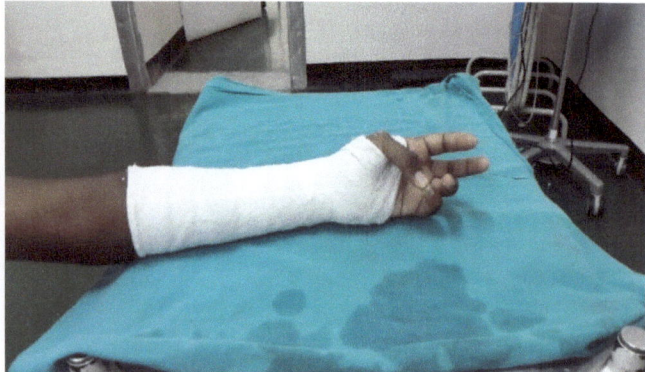

Picture 34D: Apposition of the thumb against the little finger

Note: The apposition of the thumb and/against the fingers is important

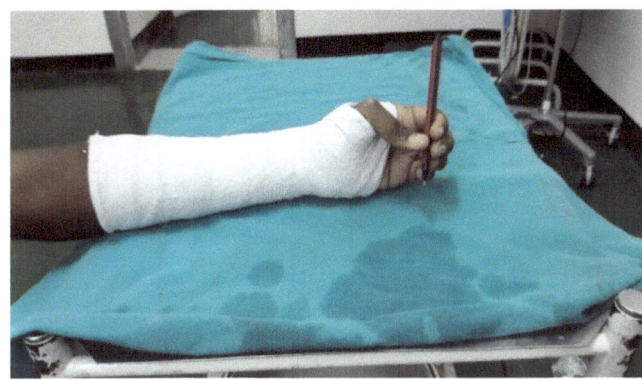 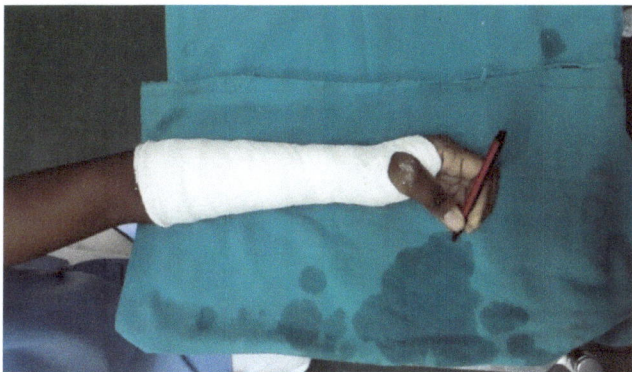

Picture 35A: Functional hand (front view) Note: The thumb's MP joint is free **Picture 35B:** Functional hand (top view)

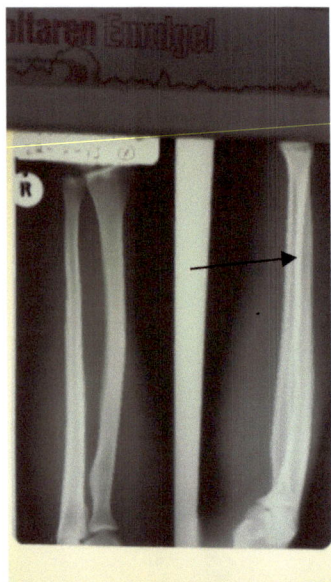 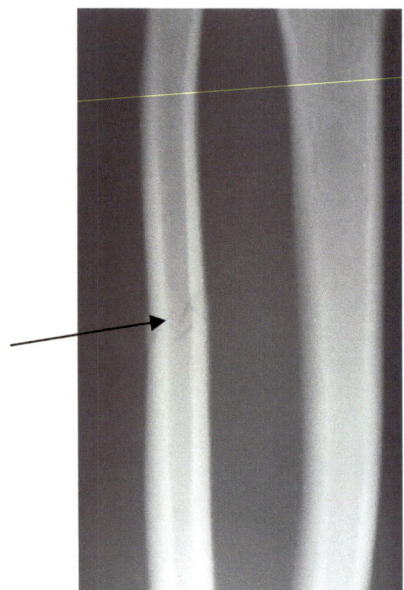

Pictures 36A – B: Fractures of the ulna shown by the arrows (Close up; Right radiograph) treated with an Above Elbow POP (see below); inappropriately

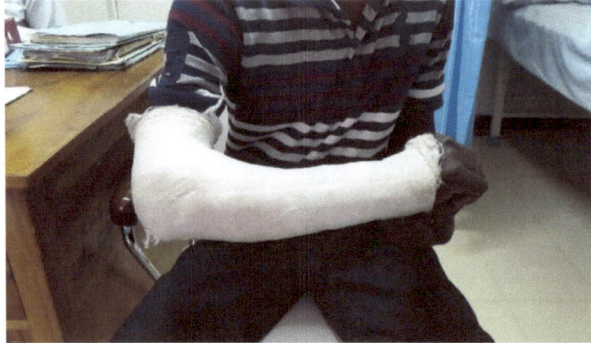

Picture 36C: Incorrectly applied "above elbow" cast for a single mid shaft ulna fracture (instead of a below elbow POP)

𝒯he preparation for the above elbow POP cast is the same as that for the below elbow POP application. The landmarks for this POP are the distal palmar crease and the level of a sergeant's budge (insertion of the Deltoid muscle). The following should be the procedure:

1. This plaster is best applied when the patient is seated with the elbow is held at 90° or more and the shoulder flexed to approximately 45-60° (anterior to the torso), held out either by the patient or an assistant. And the technician in front of the patient. This plaster can be applied with or without an assistant. If the assistant is not available, the patient can support his/her injured hand with the other uninjured limb as described above.

2. Apply the stockinet (if not available, it is not really necessary) and under-cast slightly over the intended edge of the final POP with the elbow in a functional position. The Orthopaedic wool must be wound around the elbow in a figure of 8 until the elbow is fully covered, and proceed proximally to just over the level of the sergeant's budge (insertion of the Deltoid muscle).

3. The indications for this type of POP are shown in *Table 1* above.

4. Steps 4 to 11 are similar to the steps in the above preceding procedures (as the below elbow circular cast).

Undisplaced fractures of the Humerus

Fractures of the Humerus may affect the following areas and commonly seen in various age groups:

1. Proximal metaphyseal area (The elderly)

2. The shaft (diaphysis) – young adults

3. Distal metaphyseal areas (especially in children)

Proximal Humerus

a. The head of the Humerus

b. The neck of the Humerus

c. A combination of (a) and (b) above.

There are various types of classification of such fractures. Commonly used is the Neer's classification which takes into consideration the number of pieces or main fragments resulting from the fracture. Undisplaced proximal humeral fractures are generally treated conservatively. These fractures result, usually, from low energy impact and a commonly seen in the elderly. It must, however, be emphasized that these fractures may be associated with shoulder dislocation especially if they are high energy injuries.

History and physical examination are important. Injury to the axillary nerve may be a complication of such an injury and physical evaluation of the sergeant's budge area is important. This is to evaluate the sense of feeling in the said area.

Treatment entails pain management by resting the injured limb and area; administration of analgesics and splintage. The splintage takes two forms

a) A simple collar and cuff or

b) A modified U-slab with a collar and cuff.

Note: It must be noted that long splintage periods of over six weeks, especially in the elder, must be discouraged. On the contrary, early mobilization must be encouraged to abate stiffness or shoulder ankylosis.

*I*n this chapter we hope to discuss the application of the modified U-slab. In the absence of using a U-slab, a hanging cast must be applies. The modified U-slab anchors on to the shoulder and must therefore be well molded around and above the shoulder. The modified U-slab, therefore, must be applied with attention to detail.

The Hanging cast on the other hand is applied just about the level of the fractured Humerus. It works as a weight and helps to "apply" a vertical traction onto the injured Humerus, especially when the patient is upright.

1. *Plaster of Paris Bandages – various sizes depending (appropriateness)*

2. *Under-cast material*

   a. *Stockinet (not absolutely necessary)*

   b. *Cotton wool or Orthopaedic wool bandage*

3. *Skin lotion (not absolutely necessary)*

4. *Crepe bandage*

5. *Bucket / Container*

6. *Kettle or urn*

7. *Water*

8. *A pair of POP scissors*

9. *Tape or Elastoplast to secure the undercast especially the stockinet (if available for use)*

10. *Surgical blades*

11. *Incontinent sheets and/or plaster mat (to protect the patient, linen and the floor)*

12. *Disposable gloves (may not be necessary)*

13. *Plaster or POP room / Plaster OPD-room / theatre POP room (Not absolutely necessary) can be done anywhere including the ward*

14. *Chairs or examination couch*

15. *Working surface or trolley*

16. *Apron (to protect the patient, technician and the assistant)*

17. *The injured patient*

Preparation

Prepare all the materials you plan to use before you embark on the exercise.

  a. *Estimate the number of POP bandages that will be used*
  b. *Remove the POP bandages from their plastic coverings*
  c. *Keep the POP away from water (see Figure 1 on pp 20 above)*
  d. *Make sure the water temperature is ideal*
    i. *Hot water shortens the working time while colder water prolongs the working time*
    ii. *"Dry" wet POP shortens the working time, while wetter POP prolongs working time*
  e. *Take measurements from the uninjured corresponding side of the patient (limb)*
  f. *Measure the lengths and thickness of slabs that will be used for a particular procedure beforehand*
  g. *Position the limb and patient appropriately when ready to go!*

Actual Process

1. Measure the following slabs

  a. Back-slab – from the wrist to the back of the shoulder

  b. U slab from the root of the neck; down the lateral shoulder to and around the elbow in a U fashion to the inner side (medial); short of the armpit.

  c. Posterior slab from the postero-lateral shoulder down to and just short of the elbow.

  d. Anterior slab from the antero-medial shoulder down to and just above the elbow

These slabs must be thick enough – at least 12 layers in an average adult and taken from the uninjured side (to avoid inflicting pain on the patient)

2. Measure and apply the stockinet from the hand to and above the shoulder – to the root of the neck. The arm must be in the desired position when measuring and applying the stockinet.

3. Secure the stockinet to the anterior and posterior torso (chest) with tape (or Elastoplast).

4. The patient must hold and support the injured upper limb with the sound hand by the wrist; with the elbow at 90° flexion and the shoulder in the adducted at 80° to 90°and internally rotated by the shoulder.

5. Soak the main posterior or back-slab and apply it from top (neck root) to the wrist. This is held in place by the assistant – by the shoulder and the forearm.

6. The U-slab is then soaked and applied from the neck root onto the lateral shoulder down and over the deltoid muscle toward the arm and the elbow and wound round the elbow to the medial aspect of the arm (short of the armpit).

7. The Postero-lateral and antero-lateral slabs are also applied and secured in place. All these are molded to the contours of the shoulder and arm.

8. The whole construct is secured in place with a crepe bandage from the wrist up toward the shoulder.

9. (5) to (8) above must be done swiftly to avoid the plaster of Paris from setting before molding is done properly and appropriately. It is therefore important to work with water that is cool or luke-warm (which extends the working time).

10. The assistant will be molding the antero-lateral and postero-lateral areas of the shoulder with the right and left hands respectively while facing the patient's shoulder.

11. The technician, while standing at the back of the patient, will hold and mold the proximal end near the neck root and superior part of the shoulder with his left hand; while the right hand will mold the lateral (Deltoid) area. Note that this is a patient's right shoulder.

12. The superior part of the cast will therefore "hook" on the shoulder proper so that it does not slide down the arm (toward the elbow) and in the process support the head and neck area of the Humerus.

13. Once the construct sets, the patient must be wiped clean off the undesired POP on the exposed skin.

14. The wrist is then supported in a collar and cuff and the wrist mobilization exercises are demonstrated to the patient.

These too will be managed in a similar fashion except that the construct can be removed at 4 weeks and two slabs on the lateral and medial sides of the arm (Humerus) or indeed a cylinder are applied for a further two weeks. This is to allow for early shoulder and elbow mobilization (physiotherapy). This however must be subject to clinical assessment.

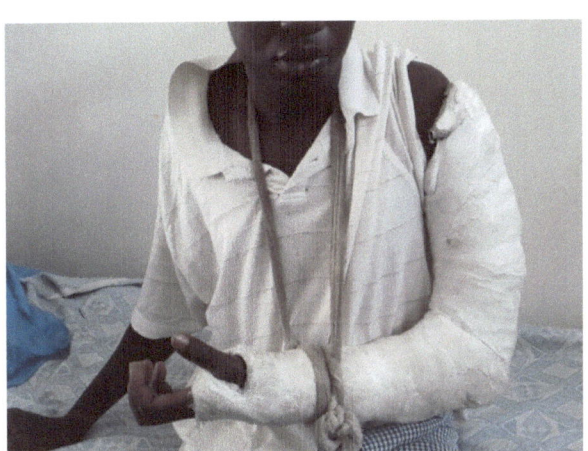

Picture 37A: Incorrectly applied POP for a left Humerus fracture

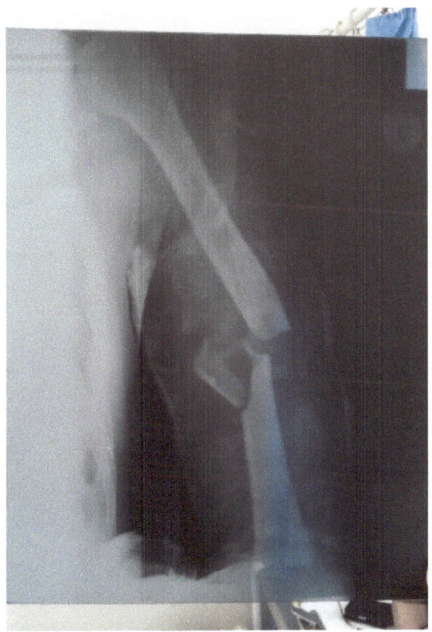

Picture 37B: Position of fracture under the cast

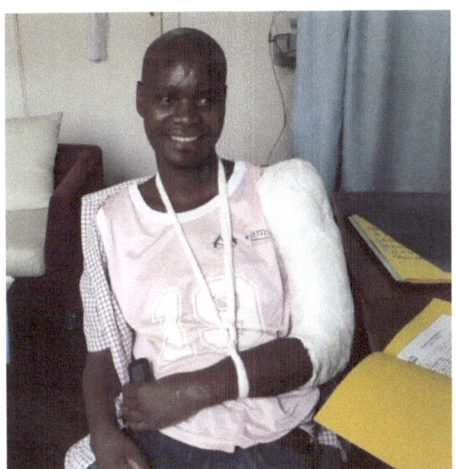

Picture 38A: Modified U-slab (Hooking on to the shoulder)

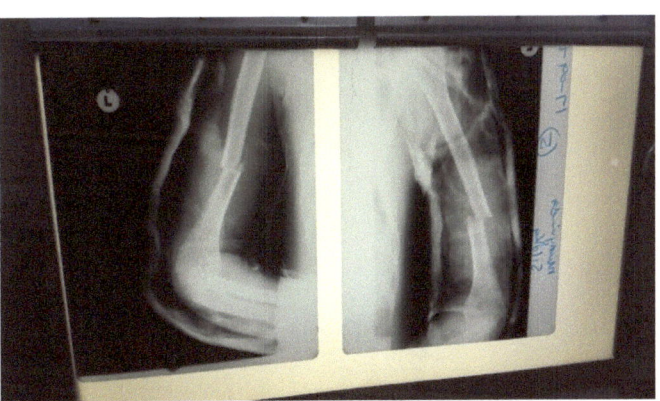

Picture 38B: Acceptable position on a "check-radiographs"

Note: Look out for the radial nerve injury in diaphyseal and diaphysio-metaphyseal humeral fractures. Check for a wrist drop before and after the application of the above said U-slab

A. Custom Made

The arm-sling is designed to support the forearm. These include the hand, forearm proper (from the wrist to the elbow). The injured forearm or/and the hand can be rested and supported in the arm-sling with or without the POP splint. These injuries include soft and/or hard tissue by whatever aetiology. The arm-sling can be factory-made or may be fashioned from a triangular bandage (*see below*).

Injuries include fractures of radius or ulna or both; wrist injuries, metacarpal bones and the fingers and soft tissue injuries of the forearm.

The arm-sling can be used for the following functions

      a. Support the forearm before splintage

      b. Support a splinted forearm; below or above elbow splintage

      c. Elevate the injured forearm whether splinted or otherwise

The arm-sling however ***must not primarily be used*** for the fracture of the Humerus on its own; unless there is another harness to strap the arm against the torso or the trunk (chest).

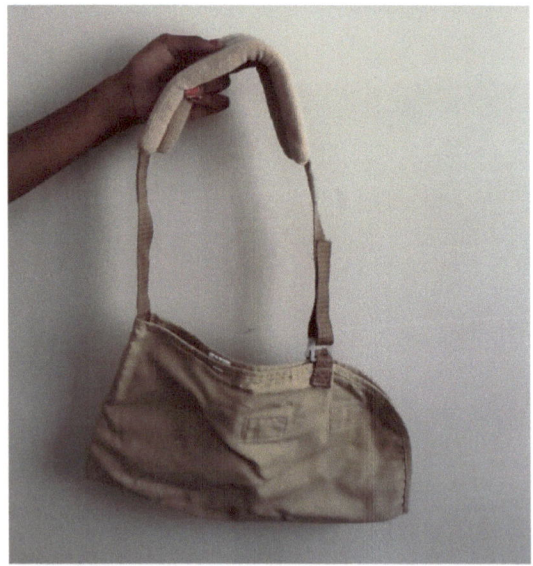

Picture 39: Custom made arm-sling

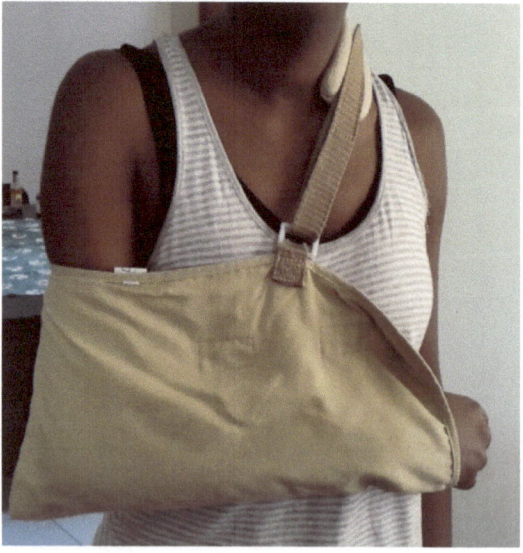

Picture 40: Forearm supported by the arm-sling

B. From a Triangular Bandage

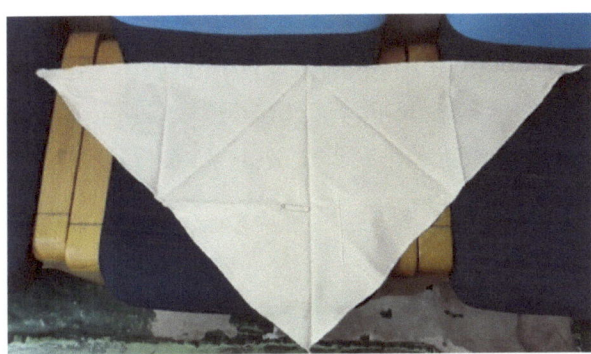

Picture 41: Triangular bandage

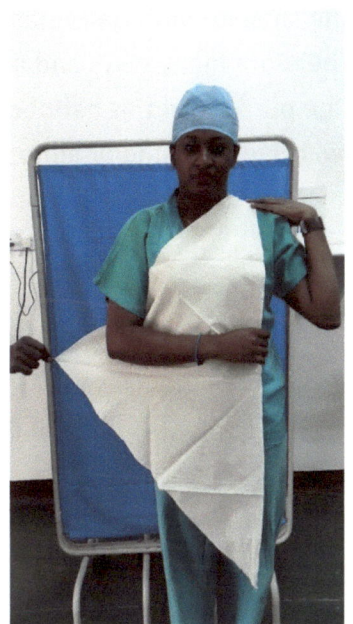

Picture 42A: Application of triangular bandage (Right arm)

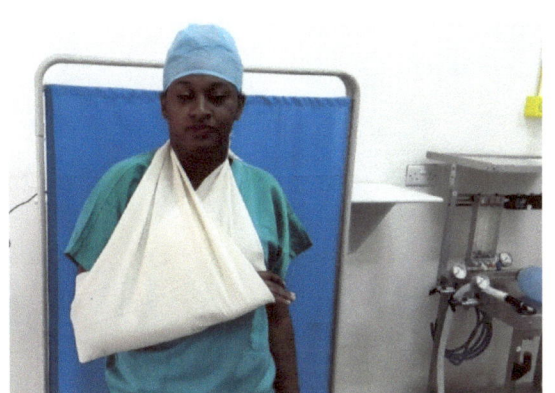

Picture 42B: Forearm & hand being supported (with mild elevation);

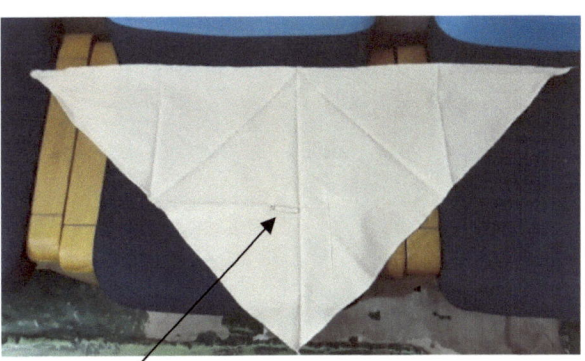

Picture 42C: Safety pin (used behind the right elbow in *Picture 42B*)

Both the collar & cuff and the arm-sling can be used for injuries around the shoulder joint and above. This would however be better if the arm is applied against the torso with a harness to rest the shoulder and clavicular area. In this case the knots must be tied on the opposite side of the injury. There are many ways and methods of securing both the arm-sling and the collar & cuff to the torso. For the purpose of this handbook and for the economically challenged countries the method describe here will give the same or almost the same level of relief required for the said injuries.

Strictly speaking the arm-sling should be called forearm sling; while the collar & cuff be called arm-sling.

A collar & cuff can be fashioned from the triangular bandage by folding it several times as illustrated below. The apex (opposite the longest length) is folded down (half the height = Ht) towards the middle of the longest length; and this is continued by folding half the remaining height until one ends up with a belt-like strap. This is the strap that will be used as the collar & cuff *(see Pictures 45 below)*.

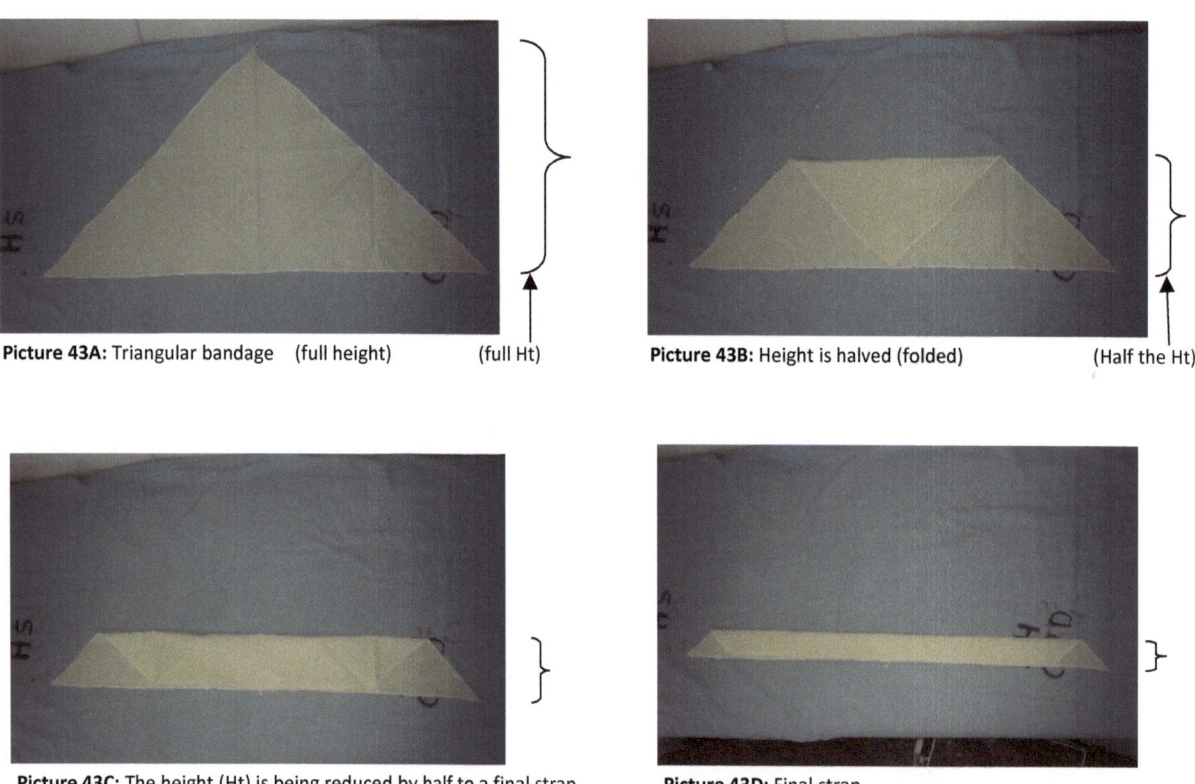

Picture 43A: Triangular bandage   (full height)   (full Ht)

Picture 43B: Height is halved (folded)   (Half the Ht)

Picture 43C: The height (Ht) is being reduced by half to a final strap

Picture 43D: Final strap

As the name suggests, the sling supports the forearm in the cuff area (wrist) and against or around the neck (collar). The collar & cuff therefore is designed and used for injuries sustained above the elbow; the shoulder and clavicular injuries. This sling too can be used to support the injured arm as well as institute elevation of the ipsilateral forearm. Caution must however be taken not to compromise the circulation to the forearm around the elbow joint. It is important therefore that the radial pulse must be looked out for and felt and palpated (equal in character and volume as on the opposite side) on the affected limb; or otherwise discontinue its use. The collar & cuff can however be applied in a forearm fracture (wrist fractures) after the fracture is under the protection of the slab or a circular cast.

A collar & cuff, however, must not be used on a freshly injured wrist as this sling will cause more damage and/or pain to the injured wrist of a patient as opposed to allowing it to rest – *this is a commonly observed misuse of the collar and cuff!!!*

See the Pictures 44A-B below

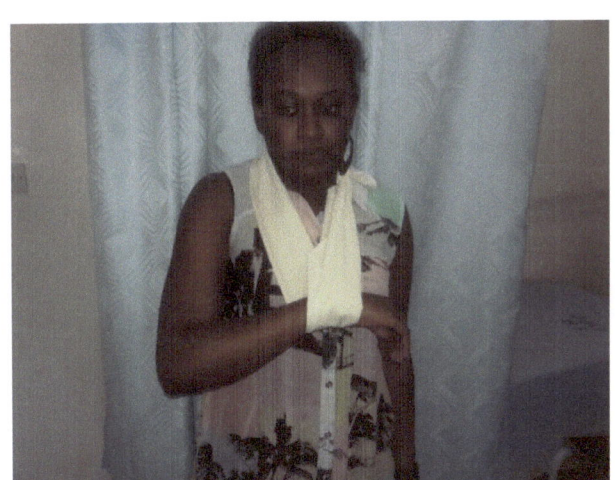 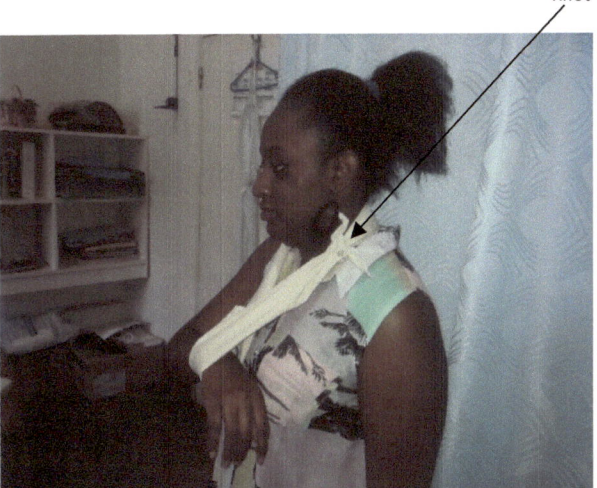

Knot

Picture 44A-B: The strap goes round the neck (Collar) and the wrist (cuff) and giving support to the Right shoulder, arm and the elbow; knot is on opposite side of the supported limb

Another type for a Collar & Cuff

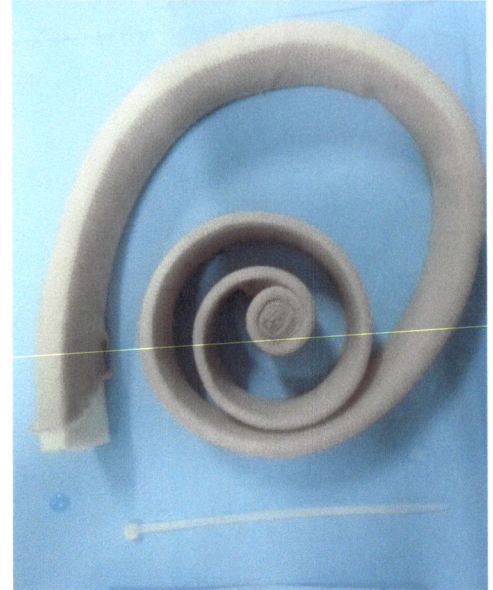

Picture 45A: Clip and mutton cloth with a soft form

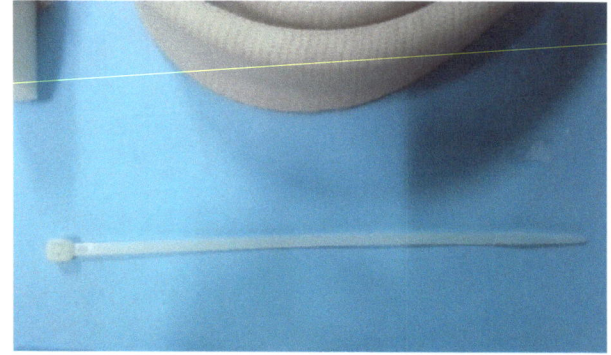

Picture 45B: Clip – close up

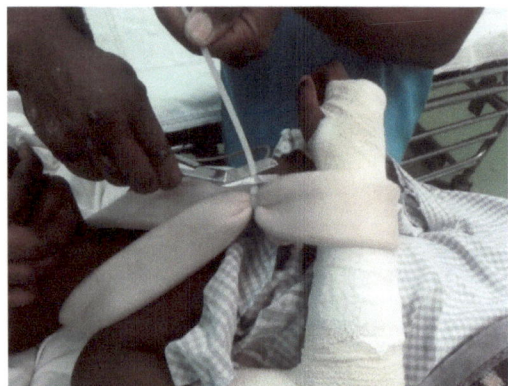

Picture 46A: Clip being cut off

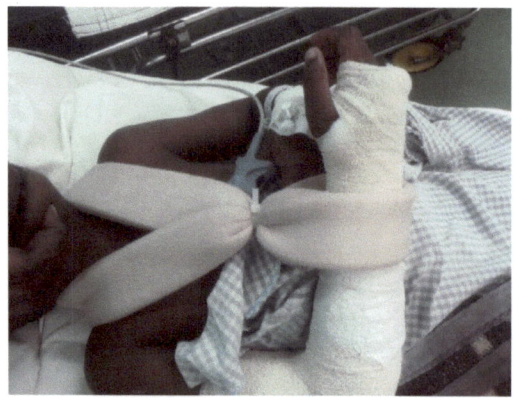

Picture 46B: Secured collar & cuff

a pillow case can easily be "modified" to offer an excellent tool for the elevation of an injured upper limb. This includes injuries of the finger, hand, wrist, and forearm.

Pick one corner of the blind or closed end of the pillow case and push it into (invaginate or in-folded into) the oppose corner on the same closed end; then the pillow will be folded into half along its length. The bottom half of the closed end can then hold the arm while the forearm will be supported inside the oblong length of the rest of the pillow case. And at the open end of the case, the rest of the pillow case will be gathered together and tied to a drip-stand with the elbow at 90°, and the shoulder at 0 to 90° abduction depending on the comfort of the patient. This can be used both in paediatric and adult patients while in supine, sitting or standing positions.

Modified Pillow Case Elevation

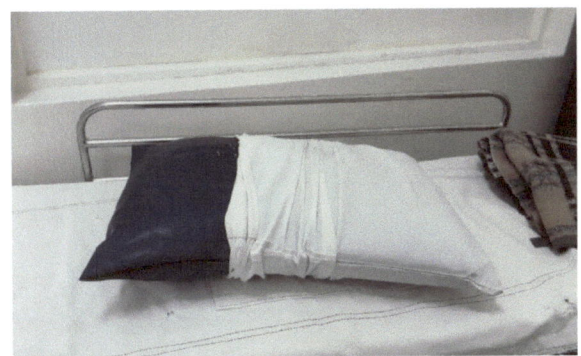

Picture 46A: Removing pillow from the case

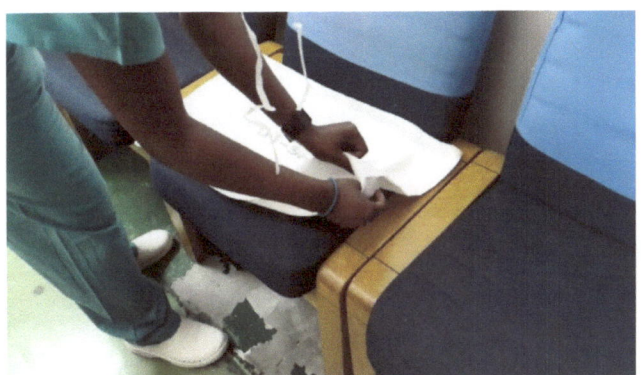

Picture 46B: Invaginating one blind corner (end) into the other

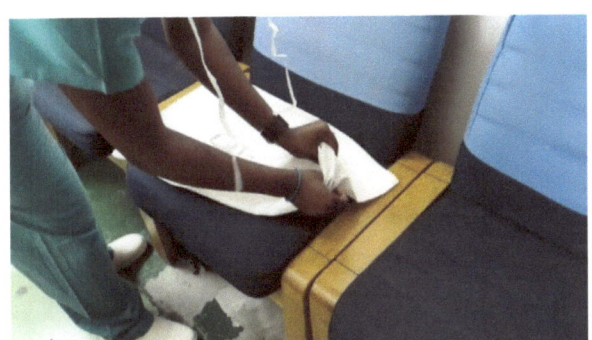

Picture 46C: Further invagination (in-folding)

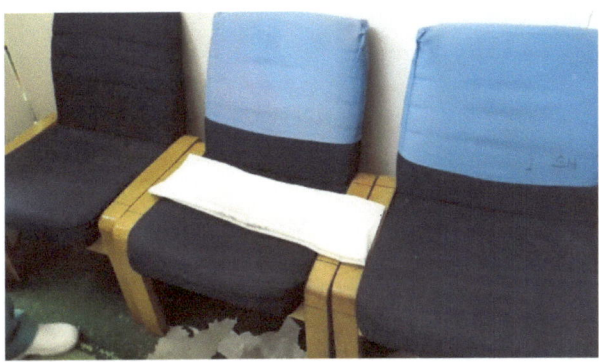

Picture 46D: Pillow case folded in half

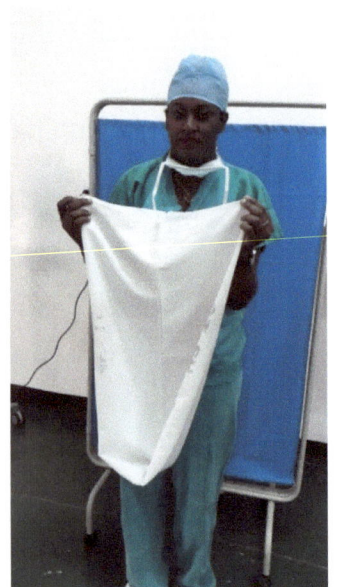

Picture 46E: Showing the pillow case pouch

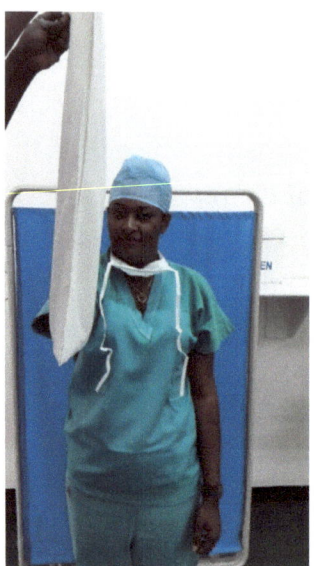

Picture 46F: Elevation of forearm with elbow & shoulder at 90°

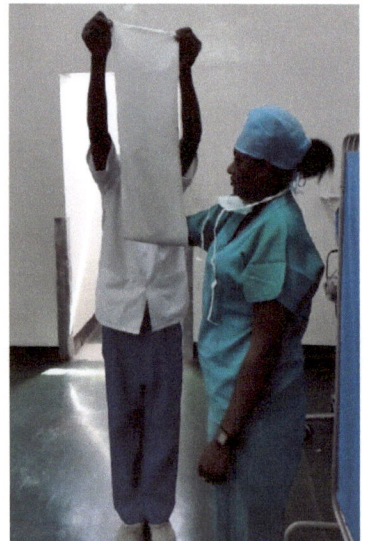

Picture 46G: Elevation in a standing posture

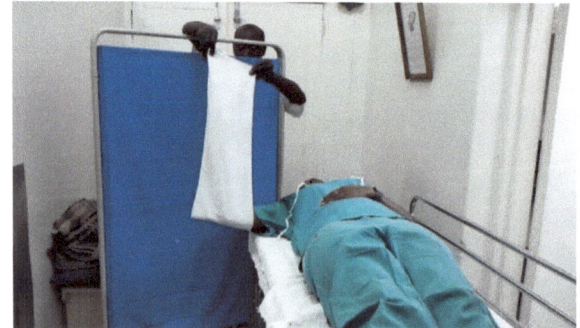

Picture 46H: Supine position with elbow and shoulder (abduction) at 90°

*𝒯*his elevation is suitable for soft and hard tissue injuries of the hand, wrist and forearm. The patient is advised to keep the hand and wrist mobile (to their level of comfort) so that the swelling in the upper limb can reduce within the shortest possible time.

Technique (details)

Preparation

The preparations for the above stated slabs are similar to the already discussed method of doing the slab in the upper limb. The slabs, both for the back and the U-slab, must be prepared beforehand. This is because they must not be done in a piece meal manner. If this is done, the first slab may set before the next is applied. The slabs therefore must be wetted and applied almost simultaneously.

The indications are the following

a) Metatarsal fractures

b) Tarsal fractures

c) Ankle sprains

d) Ankle fractures

e) Tibia or Fibula fractures

The landmarks on the foot are the metatarsal heads (distally) and four fingers below the popliteal fossa proximally. The landmarks for the below knee POP are *shown in pictures 47 A and 47 B* and the ankle joint must be at 90°as seen in *Picture A below:*

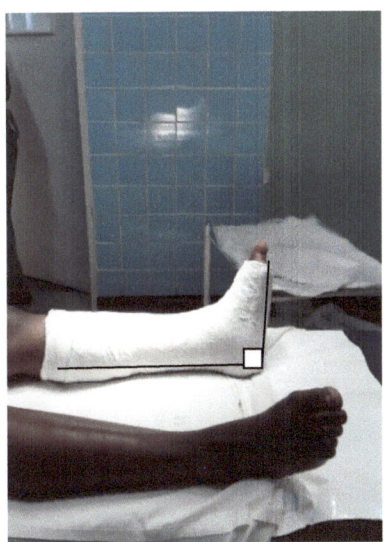
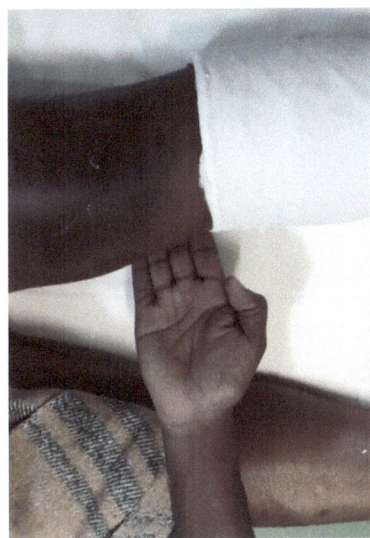
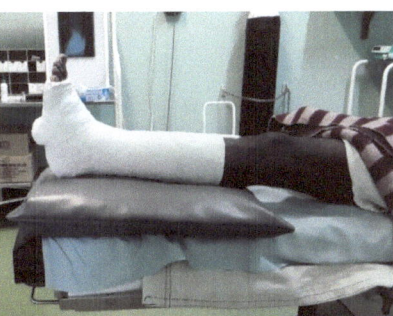

Picture47A: Ankle joint at 90°
Right foot is in equinus (natural resting position)

Picture47B: Proximal end

Picture 47C: 4-finger-breadth from popliteal fossa

Incorrect position of the ankle joint in a Plaster of Paris (for a walking below knee cast)

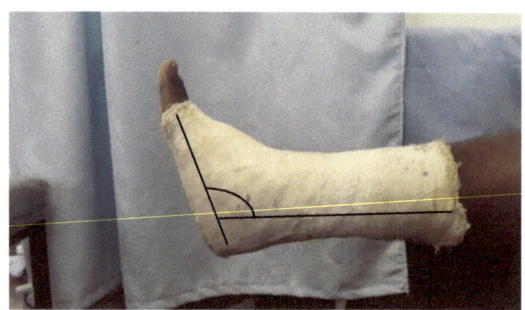

Picture 48A: Foot in equinus (medial view) more than 90°

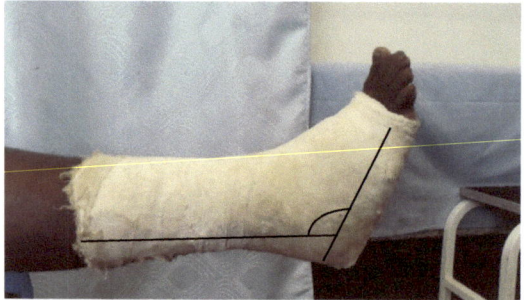

Picture 48B: Foot in equinus (lateral view) more than 90°

Note that a foot in an equinus position is in an unnatural anatomical position (for standing and walking)

Materials

The following are the materials needed to easily, effectively and efficiently apply a Plaster of Paris:

1. Plaster of Paris Bandages – various sizes depending on (appropriateness)

    a. Patient's age and built

    b. Site for application

Note: The largest/biggest size is better to have is stock as it can be cut to any appropriate size needed for the job

2. Under-cast material

    a. Stockinet

    b. Cotton wool or Orthopaedic wool

3. Skin lotion (not absolutely necessary)

4. Bucket / Container

5. Kettle or urn

6. Water

7. A pair of POP scissors

8. Surgical blades

9. Incontinent sheet and / or Plaster mat (to protect the patient, linen and the floor)

10. Disposable gloves (may not be necessary)

11. Plaster or POP room / Plaster OPD-room / theatre POP room(Not absolutely necessary) can be done anywhere including the ward

12. Chairs or examination couch

13. Linen / Pillow (may not be necessary)

14. Working surface or trolley

15. Apron (to protect the technician and the assistant)

16. The injured patient

1. The POP size is important. The slab must cover 2/3 of the circumference of the leg/foot.

2. The ankle must be plantigrade (90°)

3. The end of the crepe / cotton bandage can be secured with an Elastoplast / sticky tape or a wet strip of plaster of Paris.

4. The site of the slab is identified

5. The patient is positioned appropriately (functional position)

6. The length of the slab is measured on the uninjured side using either the Orthopaedic wool or indeed the POP bandage (to avoid causing further pain to the patient if the measurement was done on the injured side). This is done on opposite area to the injured side *with* the limb in *a functional position*. The back-slab will be measured from the metatarsal heads to 4-fingers below the popliteal fossa. This is to allow room for full flexion of the knee while the cast is on the leg. The U-slab will measure from about mid-leg on the medial side to mid-leg on the lateral side.

7. The POP bandage is then measured to the same length and width of the Orthopaedic wool that has been measured as a template and cut according to (6) above. The minimum number of layers of the slab 12 layers in children or more. This however will vary according the age, size of POP and built of a patient.

8. The required number of layers are then soaked (as a thick layer) in water. The POP "sheet" is then held in one hand over the bucket of water. The excess water is gently eased off the edges of this "sheet" of POP starting from the top downwards to drain excess water into the bucket.

9. The thick layer of POP is then laid over the pre-determined layer of Orthopaedic wool (step (6) above); and smoothened out (*avoiding wrinkles* as they are potential pressure points)

10. This is quickly lifted off the working surface (Trolley) and applied, wool against skin, onto the desired fracture site. The indication for the slabs will be according to the preamble of this chapter above.

11. The assistant(s) will hold the slabs in position while the "technician" will secure the slab using dry crepe / cotton bandage from the foot distally and cephalad(towards the head).

12. The crepe / cotton bandage must be applied in a figure of 8 over the ankle joint.

13. Once finished applying the crepe or cotton bandage, the end of the bandage is secured with either a wet strip of POP or an Elastoplast / sticky plaster.

14. The limb is then held is such a way that it is in a function position while molding the wet slab to the contours of the limb until the slab dries up or sets dry.

15. The lower limb is elevated (the foot end of the bed is elevated so that the head end is tilted downwards). The elevation helps to reduce the swelling quickly to give room for a circular cast to be applied as the subsequent definitive treatment.

16. The patient is shown the exercises to perform while the slab is in place. The patient is advised to move the toes in flexion and extension. This also improves and allows the quick reduction of the swelling but also keep the joints not involved in the injury mobile.

17. The patient is examined for any undue tenderness (pain) if/when the toes are passively extended – *to rule out the impending compartment syndrome.*

18. A patient may be discharged from the health facility on a mild analgesia and given instructions of how to look after the slab; for example, not to soak it in water; avoid sitting close to fire, to come back to the health facility especially if the pain is getting worse than before the discharge or if the slab becomes very loose that it may easily fall off the limb.

19. A review appointment date, within 48 to 72 hours, is given to the patient for removal of the slab and replacing it with a circular cast.

The Below Knee POP Circular Cast

Preparation

The preparations for the above stated circular cast are similar to the already discussed method of doing the circular cast in the upper limb. The choice, however, of size of the POP bandages for the lower limb circular casts must be appropriate to the size of the limb, both in children and adults.

This therefore means that the small-sized POP bandages must not be used on the adult's lower limb because the process of applying such a cast will be laborious, messy and of poor quality. On the converse, the large-sized POP bandage should not be used on a neonate, as it will be cumbersome to apply and will not hold well. If the latter situation is encountered, the bandage must be cut to the appropriate size to "fit" the neonatal limb size.

The following are the indications:

    a. Multiple metatarsal fractures,

    b. Tarsal fractures – e.g. Talus or the calcaneum,

    c. Ankle;

        i. Sprains

        ii. Ankle fractures –

            1. Uni-malleolar,

            2. Bi-malleolar and

            3. Tri-malleolar fractures,

    d. Tibia or Fibula fractures

The landmarks are the metatarsal heads, distally, and four fingers below the popliteal fossa proximally.

The following are the materials needed to easily and effectively apply a Plaster of Paris:

1. *Plaster of Paris Bandages – various sizes depending on (appropriateness)*

   a. *Patient's age and built*

   b. *Site for application*

Note: It is better to stock the largest/biggest size of POP bandages as it can be cut to any appropriate size needed for any other type of plaster (job)

2. *Under-cast material*

   a. *Stockinet*

   b. *Cotton wool or Orthopaedic wool*

3. *Skin lotion (not absolutely necessary)*

4. *Bucket / Container*

5. *Kettle or urn*

6. *Water*

7. *A pair of POP scissors*

8. *Surgical blades*

9. *Incontinent sheet and / or Plaster mat (to protect the patient, linen and the floor)*

10. *Disposable gloves (may not be necessary)*

11. *Plaster or POP room / Plaster OPD-room / theatre POP room (Not absolutely necessary) can be done anywhere including the ward*

12. *Chairs or examination couch*

13. *Linen / Pillow (may not be necessary)*

14. *Working surface or trolley*

15. *Apron (to protect the technician and the assistant)*

16. *The injured patient*

Preparation

Prepare all the materials you plan to use before you embark on the exercise.

   a. *Estimate the number of POP bandages that will be used*
   b. *Remove the POP bandages from their plastic coverings*
   c. *Keep the POP away from water (see Figure 1 on pp 20 above)*
   d. *Make sure the water temperature is ideal*
      iii. *Hot water shortens the working time while colder water prolongs the working time*
      iv. *"Dry" wet POP shortens the working time, while wetter POP prolongs working time*
   e. *Take measurements from the uninjured corresponding side of the patient (limb) - if applicable*
   f. *Position the limb and patient appropriately when ready to go!*

Actual Process

1. Inform the patient:

    a. Of what will be done during the process of application. And that the POP emits heat as it sets. This is to prepare the patient for that experience.

    b. The under-cast is applied from the toes and towards the knee. The under-cast must be applied slightly beyond the intended level of the final cast (metatarsal head distally and into the Popliteal fossa). These edged will then be folded back onto the required level of the cast, 4 fingers below the Popliteal fossa proximally and metatarsal heads distally. The under-cast must be applied with the ankle plantigrade without wrinkling in a motion of figure of 8. If the under-cast is applied with the foot in an equines position, the stockinet or Orthopaedic band (cotton wool) will form *wrinkles* when the foot is positioned in a plantigrade orientation during the actual POP application. These wrinkles will then become *pressure points* under the cast and may lead to decubitus ulcers (pressure ulcers) on the skin under the cast. And note that the under-cast material must be of appropriate size for the size of the leg on which it is being applied on.

2. The POP size is important as already indicated at the beginning of the chapter.

3. The ankle must be positioned at 90° as the stockinet or under-cast is being applied

4. The patient is positioned appropriately – preferably in a supine position if the "technician" has an assistant. A patient, however, can as well be in a sitting position facing the "technician", especially if the technician is applying the cast alone.

5. Analgesic medication. This may not be necessary. If a sedative is required, it should be administered a while earlier (15 - 30 minutes) before the application is undertaken. The circular cast is applied from the metatarsal heads to 4-fingers below the popliteal fossa. This is to allow, later, the patient to fully flex the knee without the POP edge "digging" into the back of the thigh which may cause ulceration.

6. Following immersion of the POP bandage into the water (as already described above), the POP application is started from the foot and cephalad towards the knee. Again, the wet POP bandage is applied is a figure of 8 around the ankle joint (just like around the elbow in the upper limb). The POP bandage must have a 50% overlap per layer. If however the POPs are in short supply, the overlap can be less to cover a larger surface area with the same length of bandage. However, the former is recommended than the latter.

7. During the actual application:

a.   One hand should hold the wet plaster bandage, while the other hand smoothens the surface where the POP has just been applied. This allows the air bubbles to escape or pushed from the under-cast and also between the layers of the wet plaster to allow it to hold as a "unit" without the onion-peel effect at the end of the procedure. This allows the POP cast to attain a firm/solid finish. The smoothening of the wet cast is clockwise or counterclockwise (in circular motions). When smoothened longitudinally/vertically or up and down, the junctions of the POP-overlaps stand out. The latter must only be done when the POP is almost set to allow for proper molding around and along the contours of the leg/foot.

b. A thick slab on the "sole" of the POP is measured and applied as such. This is to re-enforce the sole of the POP as the patient is expected to weight bear.

c. A rubber "heel" is then applied under the cast (sole of the POP foot) in the "hollow" part of the foot and not, literally, on the heel of the POP foot. This rubber heel has a rocker bottom under surface. If a rubber heel is not available, a whole small/medium sized POP bandage is soaked and secured in the same place where the rubber heel should sit. This helps in the rehabilitation and mobilization of a patient on the POP.

8. The molding is carried out evenly to follow the contours of the foot and the leg, including around and along the Tendo Achilles and the heel posteriorly.

9. The assistant(s) will hold the leg in position while the "technician" continues to mold the POP until it sets. In an event that the "technician" is a lone, the patient's forefoot (and not heel) will rest on the technician's knee with the patient's knee slightly flexed while the ankle is positioned at 90°. *The patient's foot must not rest on its heel on the technician's knee; otherwise the patient's ankle will go into an equinus orientation (position).* With the correct positioning of the foot, the technician will use both his hands to mold the POP onto the leg, ankle and foot.

10. Once the application is finished, the patient must be asked as to whether the POP is comfortable or not.

11. The lower limb is elevated (the foot end of the bed is elevated so that the head end is tilted downwards). The elevation helps to reduce the swelling quickly.

12. The patient is shown the exercises to perform while the circular cast is in place. The patient is advised to move the toes in flexion and extension. This also allows a quick and speedy reduction of the swelling and the joints (not included under the cast) to mobile.

13. The patient is examined for any undue tenderness (pain) if/when the toes are *passively extended– to rule out the impending compartment syndrome.*

14. A patient may be discharged home on appropriate walking-aids and a mild analgesia. Instructions are then given on how to look after the circular cast; for example,

    a. not to soak it in water;

    b. avoid sitting close to fire;

    c. to come back to the health facility if and/or when the pain is getting worse than before the discharge or if the circular cast becomes too loose to be effective or can easily fall off the limb.

    d. Avoid pushing objects under the POP as they attempt to scratch the itchy skin under the cast

15. A review appointment date, within 48 to 72 hours, is given to the patient for a reassessment.

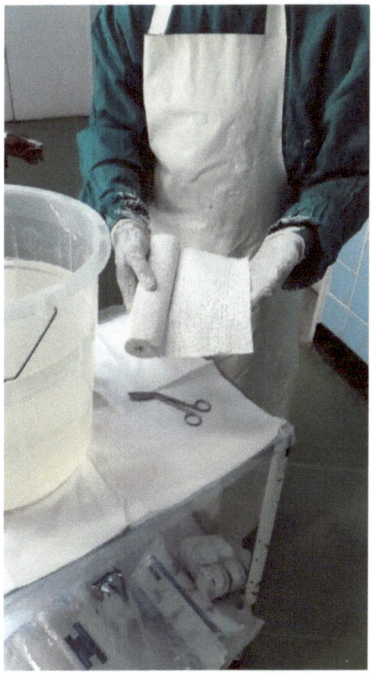

Picture 49A: Preparing to soak the POP

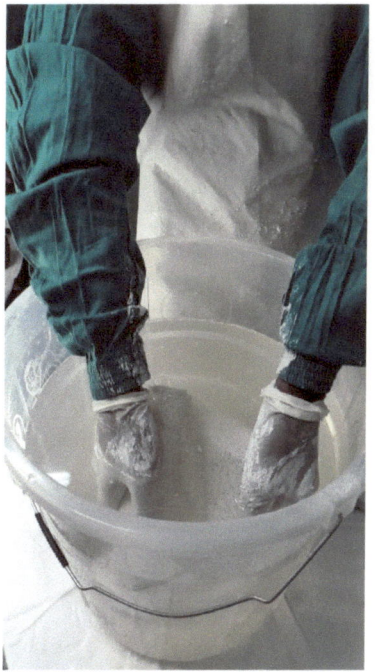

Picture 49B: Soaking the POP completely until no bubbling

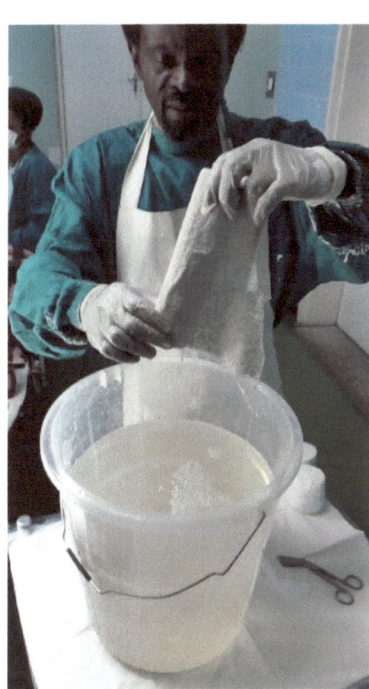

Picture 49C: Gently ease off the water from POP on one side

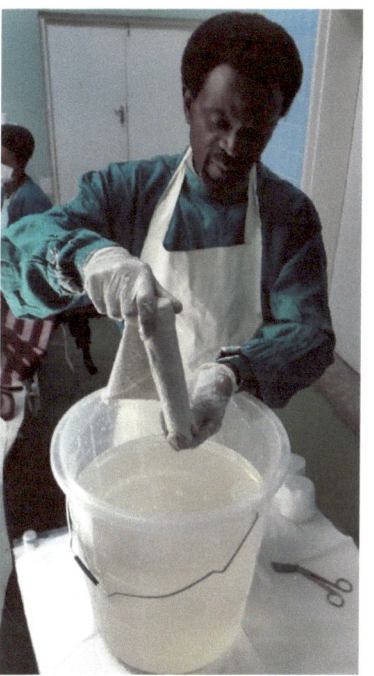

Picture 49D: Ease off water on the other side of POP end

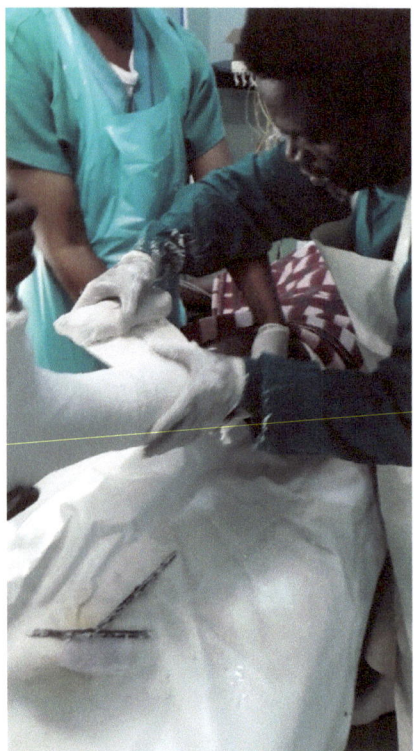

Picture 49E: Hold POP in right hand & smoothen with left

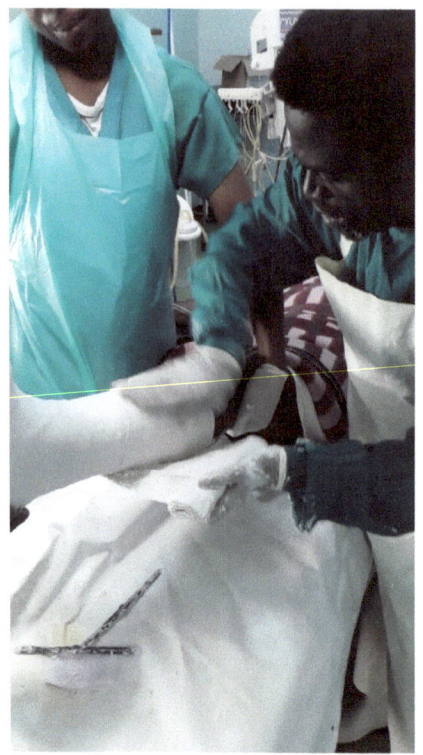

Picture 49F: Hold POP in left hand and smoothen with right

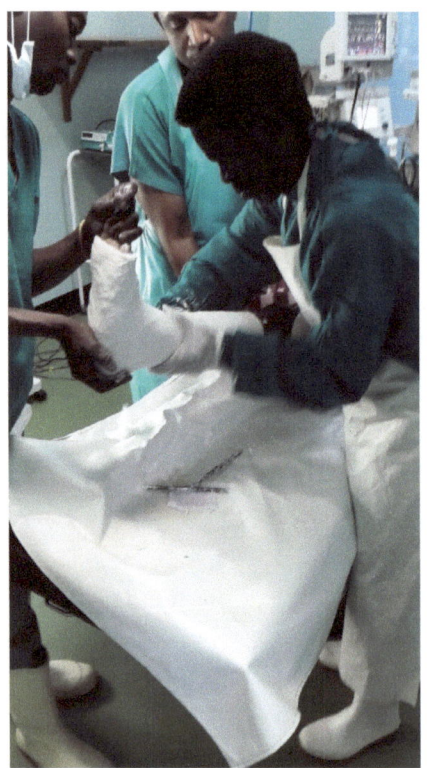

Picture 49G: Further smoothening of the below knee POP

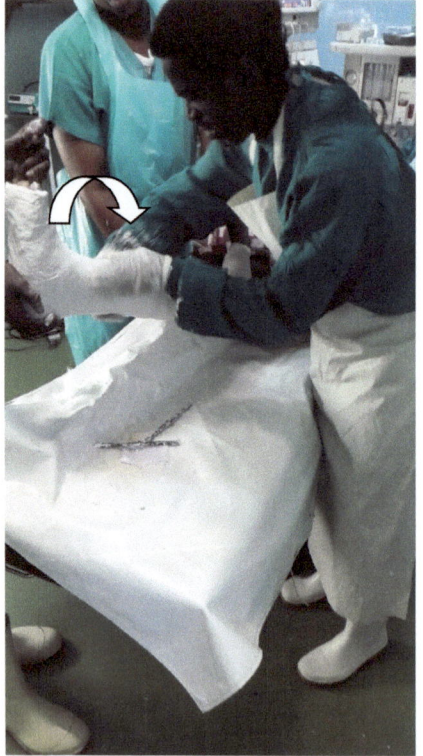

Picture 49H: Circular motion while smoothening the cast

Note Circular motions are encouraged as POP is molded to the limb. Longitudinal and firm molding pressure must be applied just before the POP sets. This is to allow the cast to take the contours of the limb

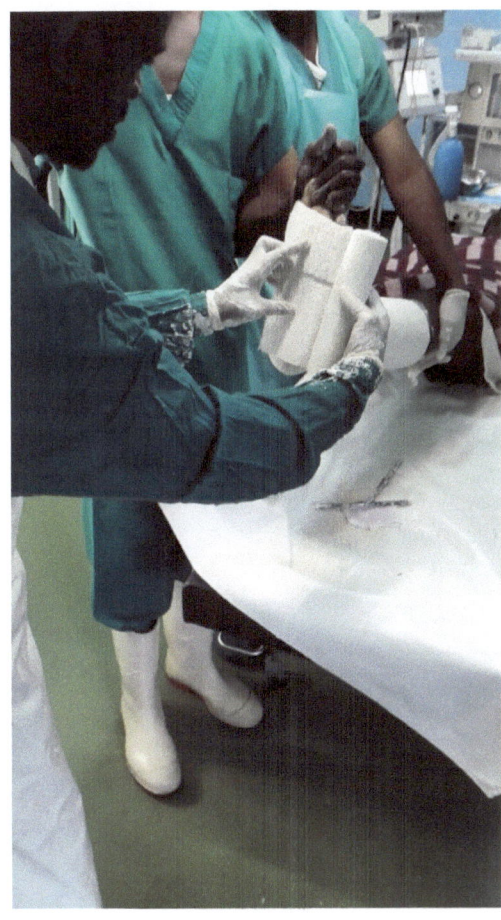

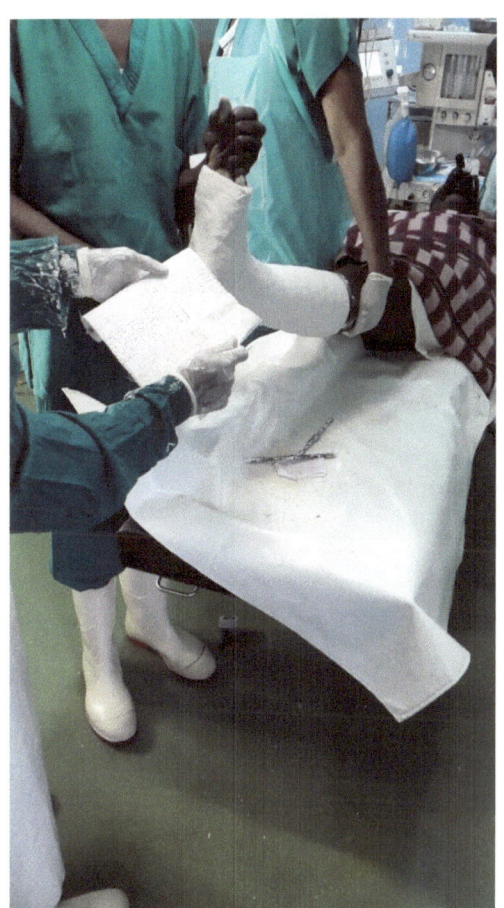

Picture 49I: Measuring the "sole" of the foot

Picture 49J: Folding the POP to form a thick "sole"

The Above Knee Back-slab

Preparation

The preparations for the above knee back-slab are similar to the already discussed method of applying the above elbow back-slab in the upper limb. The choice, however, of size of the POP bandages for the lower limb above knee casting must be appropriate to the size of the limb, both in children and adults.

This therefore means that the small sized POP bandages (5cm) must not be used on the adult's lower limb because the process of applying such a back-slab will be laborious, messy and of poor quality. On the converse, the large sized POP bandage (20cm) should not be applied on a neonate or a toddler, as it will be cumbersome to apply and will not hold well. If the latter situation is encountered, the bandage must be cut to the appropriate size to "fit" the limb of the child.

Some of the indications are the following:

a) Ligamentous knee injuries

b) Patella fracture (undisplaced)

c) Fractures of the tibia and fibula

d) Post dislocation/relocation of the knee (Look out for distal circulation!!)

e) Distal 1/3 undisplaced fracture of the femur

The landmarks are the metatarsal heads, distally, and to 4 fingers below the greater trochanter, laterally, and 4 fingers breadth from the groin medially

The following are the materials needed to easily and effectively apply a Plaster of Paris back-slab:

1. *Plaster of Paris Bandages – various sizes depending on (appropriateness)*

    a. *Patient's age and built*

    b. *Site for application*

2. *Under-cast material*

    a. *Stockinet*

    b. *Cotton wool or Orthopaedic wool*

3. *Skin lotion (not absolutely necessary)*

4. *Bucket | Container*

5. *Kettle or urn*

6. *Water*

7. *A pair of POP scissors*

8. *Surgical blades*

9. *Incontinent sheet and | or Plaster mat (to protect the patient, linen and the floor)*

10. *Disposable gloves (may not be necessary)*

11. *Plaster or POP room | Plaster OPD-room | theatre POP room (Not absolutely necessary) can be done anywhere including the ward*

12. *Examination couch | Trolley | Hospital bed*

13. *Linen | Pillow (may not be necessary)*

14. *Working surface or trolley*

15. *Apron (to protect the technician and the assistant)*

16. *The injured patient*

Technique (details)

Preparation

Prepare all the materials you plan to use before you embark on the exercise.

> a. *Estimate the number of POP bandages that will be used*
> b. *Remove the POP bandages from their plastic coverings*
> c. *Keep the POP away from water (see Figure 1 above)*
> d. *Make sure the water temperature is ideal*
>> v. *Hot water shortens the working time while colder water prolongs the working time*
>> vi. *"Dry" wet POP shortens the working time, while wetter POP prolongs working time*
> e. *Take measurements from the uninjured corresponding side of the patient (limb)*
> f. *Measure the lengths and thickness of slabs that will be used for a particular procedure beforehand*
> g. *Position the limb and patient appropriately when ready to go!*

Actual Process

1. Information to the patient:

   a. Explain what will be done during the process of application; and that the POP slab emits heat as it sets. This is to prepare the patient for that experience.

   b. The length of the slab is measured on the uninjured lower limb with the knee at 10-15° flexion and ankle at 90°. The measurement must be from 4 fingers below the greater trochanter to the metatarsal heads on the foot. The undercast may take two forms; either:

      a) A circular one between the two landmarks indicated in (1b) above or

      b) Longitudinal undercast covering 2/3 of the circumference of the limb from top-down between the indicated landmarks in (1b) above. The under-cast must be applied slightly beyond the intended level of the final cast (metatarsal head distally and proximal landmark). These edged will then be folded back onto the required level of the cast when the wet POP is finally applied and secured on the limb. It must be emphasized here that the under-cast must be applied with the ankle plantigrade (90°) and in a figure of 8 over and around the ankle area. If the under-cast is applied with the foot in an equinus position, the stockinet or Orthopaedic band (cotton wool) will form *wrinkles* when the foot is later positioned in a plantigrade orientation at the point of application. These wrinkles will then become pressure points under the securing crepe bandage and may lead to *decubitus ulcers (pressure ulcers)* on the skin. And note that the under-cast material must be of appropriate size for a particular leg.

The POP size is important as already indicated in the preceding chapters.

2. The ankle must be positioned plantigrade (90°) as the stockinet or under-cast is being applied and the knee at 10 to 15° flexion – this helps the toes to clear the ground when the patient is walking and "lock" the POP onto the knee so that the cast does not slide off the limb.

3. The patient is positioned appropriately – preferably in a supine position with the "technician" on the same side as the injured limb, with the two assistants on the opposite side holding and supporting the leg. One must hold the foot and the leg with the ankle at 90o while the other one supports the thigh with both hands with the knee flexed appropriately. The assistant on the foot-end must be in a sitting and leaning forward with his elbow resting and supported on the couch while the other hand holds the big toe of the patient and keeps the patient's ankle in position. The other assistant must remain standing while supporting the thigh. The "technician" and assistants, however, may discuss their respective positioning depending on the situation, e.g. their physique, patient size and so on.

4. Analgesic medication. This may not be necessary. If required, a sedative should be administered earlier on (about 30 minutes) before the application is undertaken (especially while and when the nurse is preparing the materials or putting materials together).

5. Following immersion of the POP slab into the water (as already described above), the POP slab application is started from the foot and cephalad towards the knee and beyond. The securing crepe or cotton bandage (wet or dry) is applied is a figure of 8 around the ankle joint (just like around the elbow in the upper limb). The crepe bandage must have a 50% overlap per layer. If however the crepe bandages are in short supply, the overlap can be less to cover a larger surface area with the same length of crepe bandage. However, the former is recommended than the latter.

6. During the actual application:

    a. If the patient's limb being applied on is big and heavy, more assistants are required as discussed in (3) above. This helps to keep the limb in the above stated functional orientation. Many hands make light work!

    b. The whole slab is soaked in water; then held on one end above the bucket of water to ease off excess water from the edges of the slab. This is done by holding the slab in one hand way above the bucket, and the other hand eases the water from the edge of the cast between the index and long fingers from top down to the bottom. Then the reverse is done with the other hand holding the top part, while the opposite index and long fingers will ease the water off the other edge into the bucket or dish. Alternatively, if the length is too long, the POP slab is crumpled and squeezed between the two hands over the bucket of water while holding the two ends

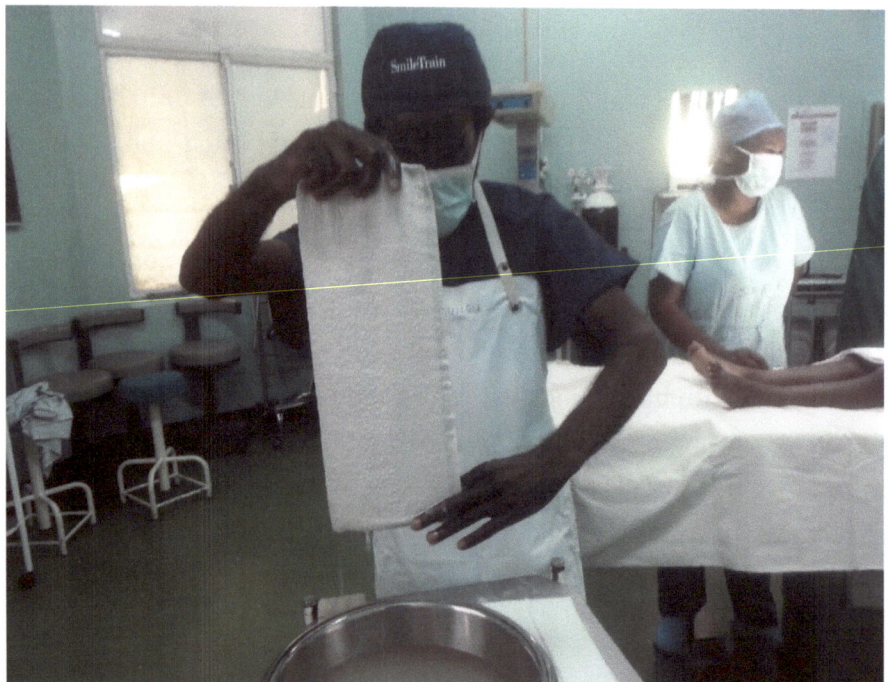

Picture 50: Gentle easing water off the POP slab edge between the left index and long fingers

    c.   The slab is then applied onto the padded limb; starting from the foot and proceeding proximally, way above the knee. This is done with the help of the assistants on a correctly positioned limb.

7. The slab is then secured with a wet or dry crepe (cotton) bandage. The molding is carried out evenly following the contours of the foot, the leg, the knee and the thigh including around and along the Tendo Achilles and the heel posteriorly.

8. The assistant(s) will hold the leg in position while the "technician" continues to mold the POP until it sets. In an event that the "technician" is a lone, (s)he must call for help before embarking on applying the cast and "educate" the helpers on what and how they must assist him/her; and also guide them during the actual process of applying the slab. This is as regards the knee and ankle angulations, soaking of the slab and actual application onto the patient's limb.

9. Once the slab application is complete, the patient must be asked as to whether they feel comfortable within the POP back-slab or not; if it is done under anaesthesia, the patient will be asked as soon as they recover from anaesthesia.

10. The lower limb is elevated (the foot end of the bed, is elevated so that the head end is tilted downwards). The elevation helps to reduce the oedema in the swollen limb quickly.

11. The patient is shown the exercises to perform while the back-slab is in place. The patient is advised to move the toes into flexion and extension. This also helps to further quicken the

reduction of the swelling but also keep the joints that are not enclosed in the slab, to be mobile.

12. The patient is examined for any undue tenderness (pain) if/when the toes are *passively extended – to rule out the impending compartment syndrome!*

13. A patient may be discharged home appropriate walking aids via the physiotherapy department. A mild analgesia may be prescribed and instructions on how to look after the slab also given; for example:

    a. not to soak POP back-slab in water;

    b. avoid sitting close to fire with the back-slab;

    c. to come back to the hospital if and or when the pain become worse than before the discharge or if the slab becomes too loose that it is not effective or may easily fall off the limb

    d. The patient may be referred to another center with the slab for further management if or when it when it is necessary.

14. A review appointment date, within 48 to 72 hours, is given to the patient for a reassessment and definitive treatment with a circular cast.

15. If the patient is on the ward, a reassessment is done within 48-72hours and a definitive circular cast applied before allowing the patient home. The patient must not apply weight on the cast until the subsequent circular cast cures within next 36 hours.

Note: That too tight a back-slab cast may/will lead to complications.

Preparations

The preparations for the above stated circular cast are similar to any circular cast. The choice, however, of size of the POP bandages for the lower limb circular casts must be appropriate to the size of the limb, both in children and adults.

This therefore means that the small sized POP bandages (3.5 or 5cm) must not be used on the adult's lower limb because the process of applying such a cast will be laborious, messy and often result in a poor quality cast. On the contrary, the large sized POP bandage should not be applied on a neonate or a toddler, as it will be cumbersome to apply and will not hold well. If the latter situation is encountered, the bandage must be cut to the appropriate size to "fit" the limb of the child.

Some of the indications are the following:

c) Tibia and fibula fracture on the ipsilateral side (in the same leg or on the same side)

d) A high tibia fracture (in the proximal 1/3)

   1. Tibial plateau fracture – undisplaced

      a. Uni-plateau

      b. Bi-plateau

e) Neck of fibula fracture

f) Torn ligaments around the knee

g) Post knee dislocation – secondary application (*look out for distal limb blood circulation!!!*)

h) Undisplaced patella fracture

i) Distal undisplaced femur fracture

   1. Within distal 1/3

   2. Condylar femoral fractures

Note: The landmarks are the metatarsal heads, distally, and about half or ¾ of the thigh above the knee proximally

Materials

The following are the materials needed to easily and effectively apply a Plaster of Paris:

1. Plaster of Paris Bandages – various sizes depending on (appropriateness)

    a. Patient's age and built

    b. Site for application

2. Under-cast material

    a. Stockinet (not absolutely necessary)

    b. Cotton wool or Orthopaedic wool

3. Skin lotion (not absolutely necessary)

4. Bucket / Container

5. Kettle or urn (to heat the water)

6. Water

7. A pair of POP scissors

8. Surgical blades

9. Incontinent sheets and/or plaster mat (to protect the patient, linen and the floor)

10. Disposable gloves (may not be necessary)

11. Plaster or POP room / Plaster OPD-room / theatre POP room (Not absolutely necessary) can be done anywhere including the ward

12. Examination couch / Trolley / Hospital bed

13. Linen / Pillow (where applicable)

14. Working surface or trolley

15. Apron (to protect the technician and the assistant)

16. The injured patient

Preparation

Prepare all the materials you plan to use before you embark on the exercise.

> a. *Estimate the number of POP bandages that will be used*
> b. *Remove the POP bandages from their plastic coverings*
> c. *Keep the POP away from water (see Figure 1 above)*
> d. *Make sure the water temperature is ideal*
>> vii. *Hot water shortens the working time while colder water prolongs the working time*
>> viii. *"Dry" wet POP shortens the working time, while wetter POP prolongs working time*
> e. *Take measurements from the uninjured corresponding side of the patient (limb)*
> f. *Position the limb and patient appropriately when ready to go!*

Actual Process

1. Inform the patient:

   a. Explain what will be done during the process of application; and that the POP emits heat as it sets. This is to prepare the patient for that experience.

   b. The patient is positioned in a supine orientation (facing upwards). The limb is held in the required position by the assistant(s), as indicated below. The under-cast is applied from the toes towards the thigh. The under-cast must be applied slightly beyond the intended level of the final cast. The upper limit of the POP must be 4-finger-breath from the greater trochanter and 4-finger-breath from the groin. These edges will then be folded back onto the required level of the cast. The under-cast is applied with a 50% overlap so as to have a-two-layer padding on the limb. The under-cast must be applied with the ankle plantigrade (at 90°) without wrinkling, in a figure of 8 maneuvers and with the knee flexed between 10 to 15°. This is important for the patient to be able to clear the ground as (s)he is walking in the cast during the rehabilitation. Remember that the natural position of the foot in a person lying in a supine position will be in equinus. And if, therefore, the under-cast is applied with the foot in an equinus position, the stockinet or Orthopaedic wool (cotton wool) will form *wrinkles* when the foot is positioned into a plantigrade orientation at the time of applying the POP. *These wrinkles will then become pressure points under the cast and may lead to decubitus ulcers (pressure ulcers) on the skin on the anterior surface of the ankle.* And note that the under-cast material must be of appropriate size for the size of the leg it is being applied on.

2. The POP size is important as already indicated in the earlier chapters.

3. The ankle must be positioned plantigrade (90°) as the stockinet or under-cast is being applied

4. The patient is positioned appropriately – in a supine position and the limb held by assistants.

5. Analgesic medication. This may not be necessary. If, however, it is required a sedative should be administered at least 15 to 30 minutes in advance before the application is undertaken. The circular cast is applied from the metatarsal heads to the level indicated above. During the application, it is important that the assistants keep the patient's limb with the joints (the ankle and the knee) in the desired position; which means the hip will be in a slightly flexed position as the leg will be off the couch. The assistant should therefore be on the opposite side of the couch facing the "technician" who will be applying the cast. One of the assistants might find it comfortable to be seated with one of his elbows supported firmly onto the couch while the other hand will be holding the foot (holding and maintaining the ankle position) by the patient's big toe. The other assistant holds the thigh with both hands while the knee is flexed. The affected limb will therefore be off the couch – this is for ease clearance or passage of the Orthopaedic wool and indeed the POP bandage under the leg as the technician applies the cast. *Note that the hand that is holding the foot must not place the patient's foot into equinus, dorsiflexion, inverted or everted*

6. Following immersion of the POP bandage into the water (as described already above), the POP application is started from the foot and cephalad towards the knee. Again, the wet POP bandage is applied is a figure of 8 motion around the ankle joint (just like around the elbow in the upper limb). The wet POP bandage must have a 50% overlap per layer. If however the POPs are in short supply, the overlap can be less than 50% to cover a larger surface area with the same length of bandage. The former, however, is recommended than the latter. Note that the application of the subsequent wet POP bandage should start where the last one ended. This allows for an evenly applied cast from the foot to the thigh and vice versa.

7. During the actual application:

    a. One hand of the "technician" should hold the wet plaster bandage, while the other hand smoothens the surface where the POP has just been applied. This allows the air bubbles to be pushed out and escape from the under-cast as well as between the layers of the wet plaster and allow the cast to set a "unit" without the "onion layer effect" at the end of the procedure. This therefore allows the POP cast to attain a firm/solid finish. The smoothening of the wet cast is clockwise or counterclockwise in a circular motion. When smoothening is done on a wet POP bandage, longitudinally/vertically or up and down, the junctions of the overlaps stand out. The latter should only be done when the POP is almost set to allow for proper molding around the foot, ankle, Achilles tendon and the knee; as well as along the contours of the leg (shin).

    b. A thickened sole slab is designed to fit the foot. This is to prepare for the wear and tear that is anticipated on the sole of the POP during rehabilitation.

c. A rubber "heel" is then applied under the cast (sole of the POP foot) in the "hollow" part of the foot (mid-foot) and not on, literally, the heel of the POP foot. This rubber heel has a rocker bottom under surface. This design of the rubber heel allows the foot in the cast to "roll" over when the patient is walking on it. If a rubber heel is not available, a whole small/medium sized POP bandage is soaked and secured in the same place where the rubber heel would/should sit. As earlier stated this helps in the mobilization of a patient on the POP.

8. The molding is carried out evenly to follow the contours of the foot and the leg, including around and along the Tendo Achilles and the heel posteriorly, about the knee and all the way up proximally.

9. The assistant(s) will hold the leg in position while the "technician" continues to mold the POP until it sets.

10. Once the application is completed, the patient must be asked as to whether the POP is comfortable or not.

11. The lower limb is then rested on an oblong pillow to allow for the POP to set solidly. This circular cast will be applied on a limb than is not in danger to further swelling (oedema).

12. The patient is shown the exercises to perform while the circular cast is in place. The patient is advised to move the toes into flexion and extension. This also helps the further reduction of the swelling but also increases the rate of healing in the limb. The toes that not enclosed in the cast are allowed to mobile as they are not part of the area of injury.

13. The patient is re-examined for any undue tenderness (pain) if/when the toes are *passively extended; this is to help to rule out the impending compartment syndrome.*

14. The patient is shown how to use the crutches (axillary or elbow) by the physiotherapist with non-weight bearing on the casted limb. This is to allow the POP to cure within 48 to 72 hours.

15. A patient may be discharged home on a mild analgesia and given instructions on how to look after the circular cast; for example,

    a. Not to soak it in water;

    b. Avoid sitting close to fire;

    c. To come back to the health facility if and/or when the pain is becoming worse off than before the patient's discharge; or if the circular cast becomes too loose that it is not effective or can easily fall off the limb

    d. If the cast has developed cracks

e. A painful area away from the injury site. It may be a decubitus ulcer (pressure sore) developing. The patient must report back to the hospital immediately.

f. Or any other concerns by and from the patient.

g. Avoid pushing foreign objects in between the skin and the POP in an attempt to scratch

16. A review appointment date, within 48 to 72 hours, is given to the patient for a reassessment.

There are various, including ingenious, ways of effecting the elevation of the injured lower limbs while patient is in bed. It must be mentioned here that a pillow or in deed pile of pillows may be used to elevate a lower limb. It, however, takes the educating of the patient and the staff about this, and close monitoring or supervision of the patient by the attending nurses (and doctors) to see that the limb is properly elevated. The pillow elevation is usually ineffective, especially, when the patient is sleeping as the limb may "fall" off the pillow. It is therefore important to institute measures that will allow prudent lower limb elevation at all times.

Some of these methods are shown below by the photographs.

It must be noted that elevation is more effective when the injured limb is elevated above the level of the heart. While the limb is in this position, the patient must be encouraged to actively (or passively) move the toes and the ankles (fingers and the wrist in upper limbs) to easily and quickly reduce the oedema in the affected injured limb. Isometric exercises are also encouraged (this is the tensing and relaxing of muscles about a joint without the movement of the particular joint). Early reduction in the oedema of a limb will help in reducing the hospital stay and early application of the required final cast; or whatever the situation may dictate.

Active mobilization of the toes, muscles about ankle (fingers and wrist) under a POP cast produce isometric exercises which improve and promote increased blood supply (perfusion) to the injured limb and further enhances healing.

Elevation of an injured limb

Lower limb

Different methods of elevating the injured lower limb

Some of the correct and incorrect methods of elevating the lower limb

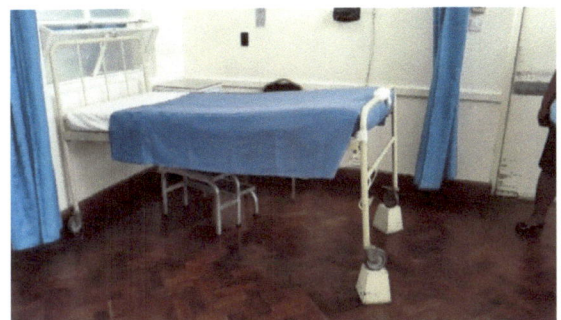

Picture 51A: Side view – showing elevation of foot-end of the bed

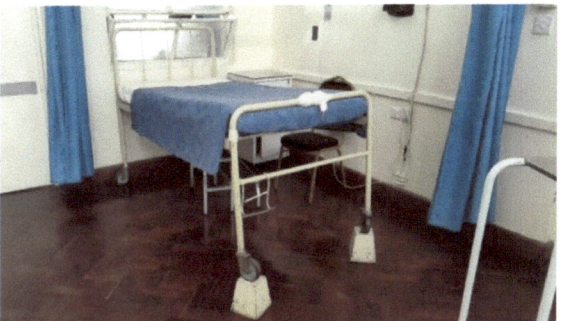

Picture 51B: Oblique view – showing elevation with blocks

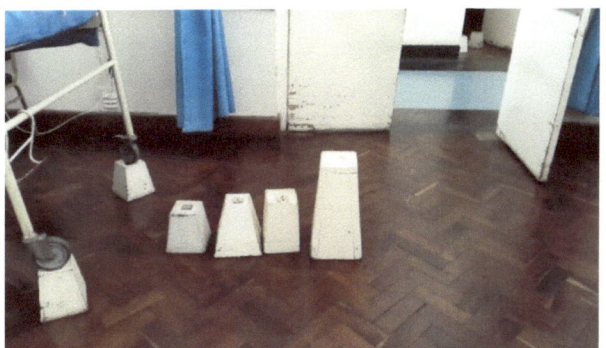

Picture 51C: A variety of blocks can be used for a desired level of elevation

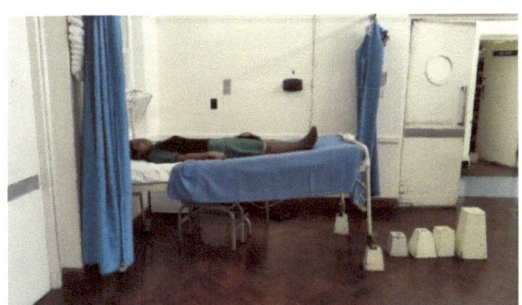

Picture 51D: Correct: Elevation using blocks – with knees in full extension

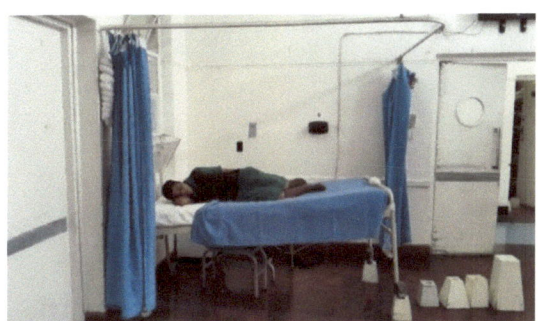

Picture 51E: Correct: Elevation despite knees being flexed

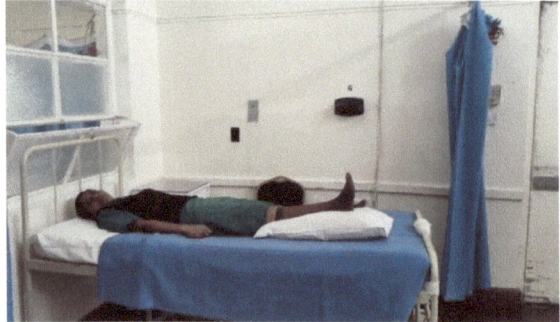

Picture 52A: Correct: Elevation of right lower limb on a pillow

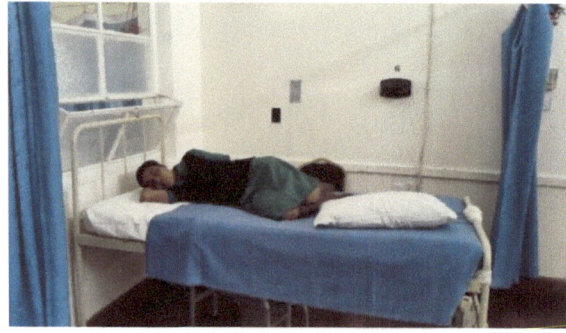

Picture 52B: Incorrect: When lower limbs are flexed; elevation is lost

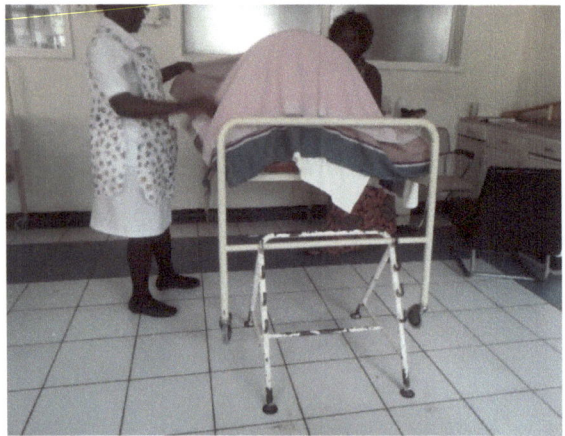

Picture 53A: Correct: Using the "A-frame" – front view

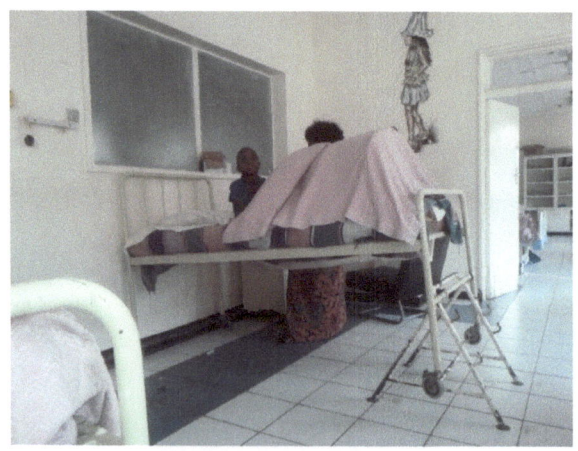

Picture 53B: Correct: "A-frame" from side view

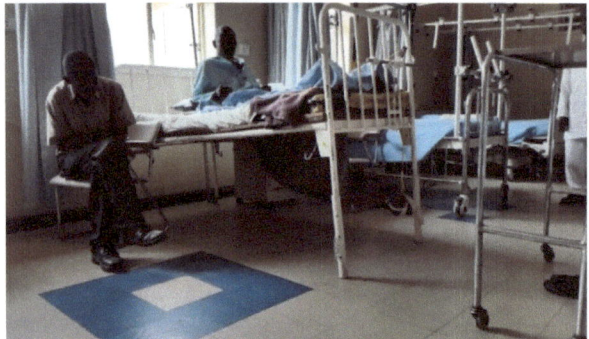

Picture 54A: Correct: Adjustable foot-end bed "legs"

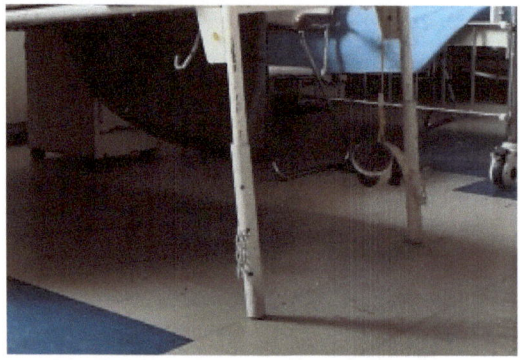

Picture 54B: Close up of adjustable foot-end bed "legs"

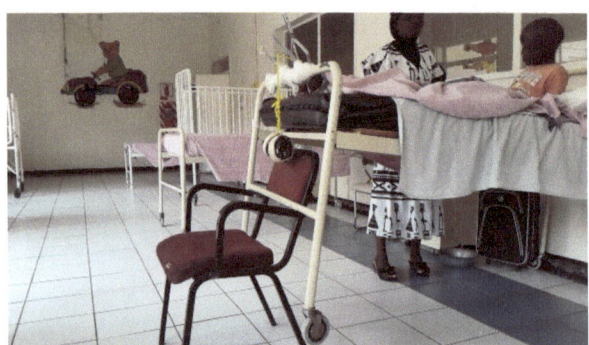

Picture 55: Correct: Using a chair

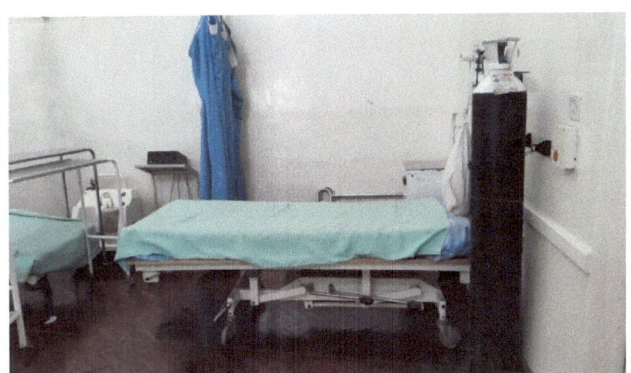

Picture 56A: Bed with in-built tilting mechanism

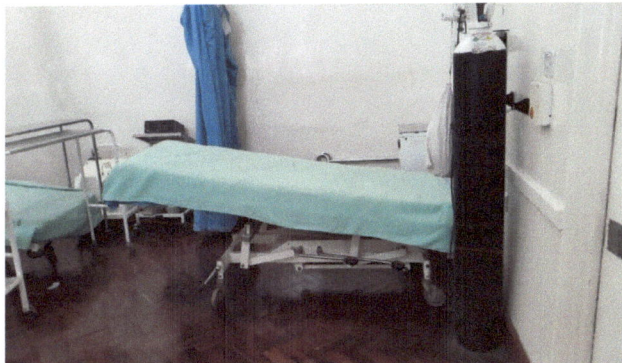

Picture 56B: Elevation of Foot-end of the hospital bed

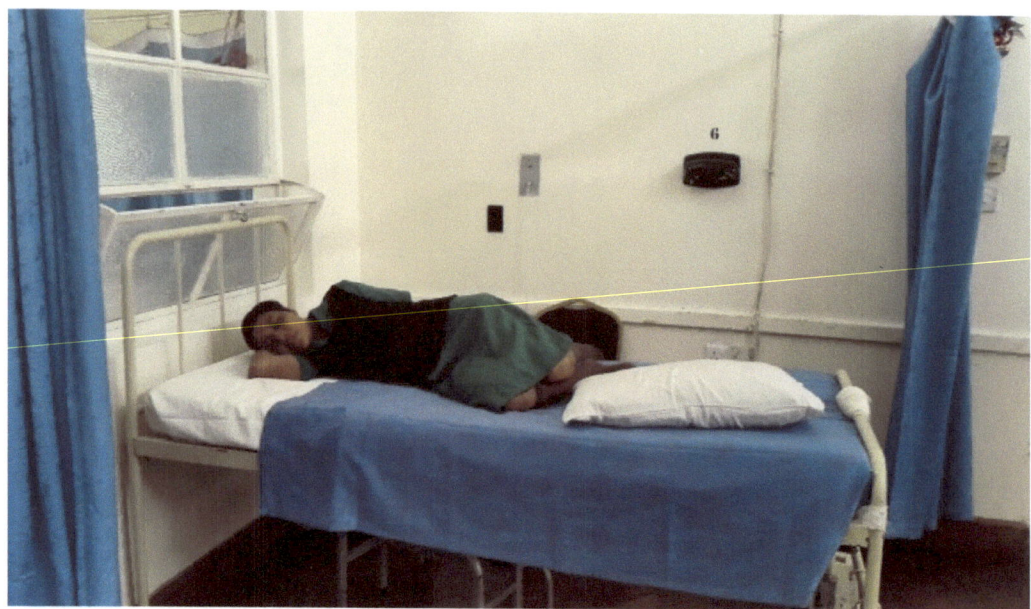

Picture 57: A pillow may be used for lower limb elevation but must be monitored closely

*P*laster of Paris takes approximately 36 hours to cure (harden). It is therefore important that we know how to dispose of the water in which POP bandages was being soaked.

It is advisable not to dispose of the Plaster of Paris through a regular hand-washing basin with the regular drainage piping. The waste must be disposed off in a large bore drainage pipe – this is to avoid the Plaster of Paris blocking the drainage pipes especially if that pipe is in the designated POP application room.

The drainage pipes must therefore be purpose designed.

Upper limbs

*L*istening to and clinical examination of a patient are the ultimate hallmark of patient care. It is therefore important to listen, observe and examine the behavior of the patient; especially a child who is in a POP cast.

If a child with a forearm fractured limb and in a cast "shakes" hands with a stranger (a doctor or otherwise) using the same injured limb (which is in a cast); the fracture on that limb is most probably healed. However, the empirical periods to fracture healing are indicated below.

A cast should be on a child's upper limb for 3 to 4 weeks and 6 to 8 weeks on an adult. The assessment of fracture healing however must be established at the earliest time (3 weeks in children) and 6 weeks in adults. This is done clinically; if the patient (child or adult) is able to exert pressure or tension on the limb under the cast and there is no sign of tenderness, this is an indication that the fracture has clinically united.

Age	Upper Limbs	Lower limbs
Children	3 – 4 weeks	6 – 8 weeks
Adults	6 - 8weeks	12 – 15 weeks

Table 2: Showing empirical fracture healing periods

Before the cast is removed, a clinical examination for union is done. If there is tenderness at the fracture site, the fracture is not healed. In that case, an extension of time is availed to the patient to be in the cast. If however, the fracture shows union under the cast, the POP can then be removed and the limb is re-examined for clinical union again and radiological union if the facilities for radiological examination are available.

Note that, at this stage any joint adjacent to the fracture site which was under the cast may exhibit signs of tenderness or pain (due to impending/ensuing stiffness). The patient may therefore complain of pain in the joint and *not* at the fracture site. This is largely due to stiffness or ensuing stiffness in the adjacent joint. It is therefore imperative to explain to the patient, or indeed the guardian to the patient.

When out of the cast joint mobilization and later strengthening of muscle are embarked on through the physiotherapy department. The patient is then followed up in the appropriate clinic or Out Patient Department until discharge from the health facility.

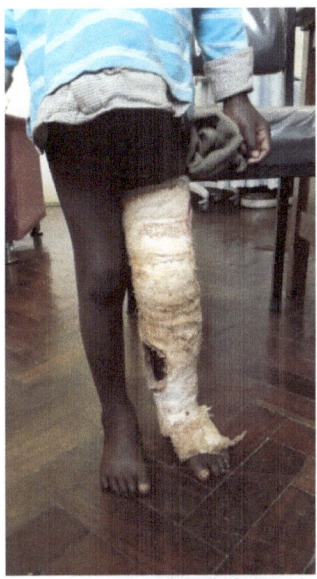

Picture 58A: Worn "sole" of above knee POP in a child

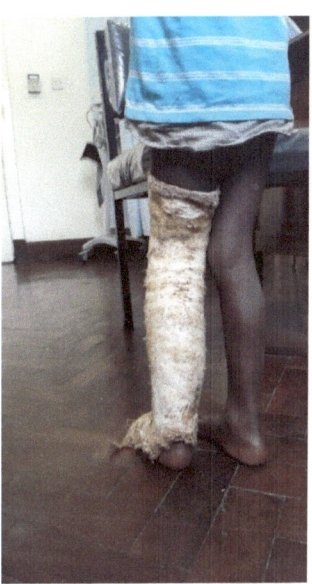

Picture 58B: Worn "sole" of POP in a child

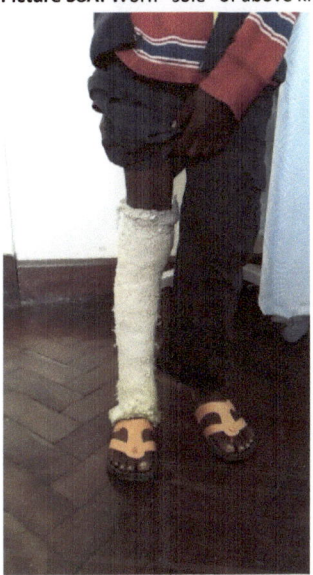

Picture 58C: Another worn "sole"

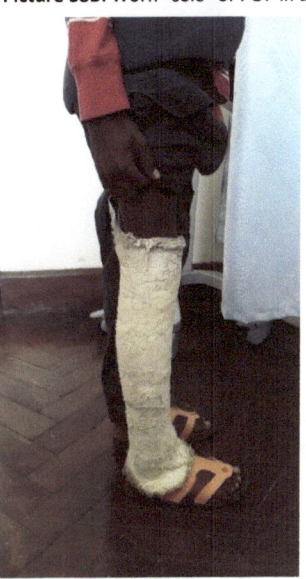

Picture 58D: Side view

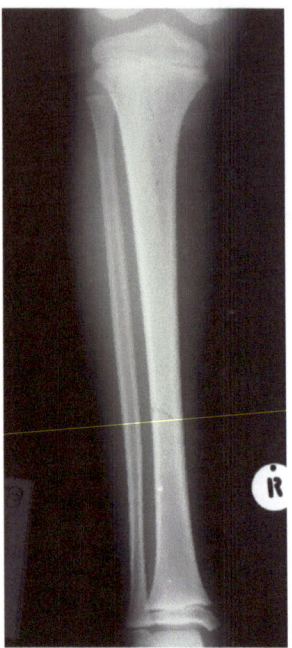

Radiograph - AP view: child in Pictures of 58C-D

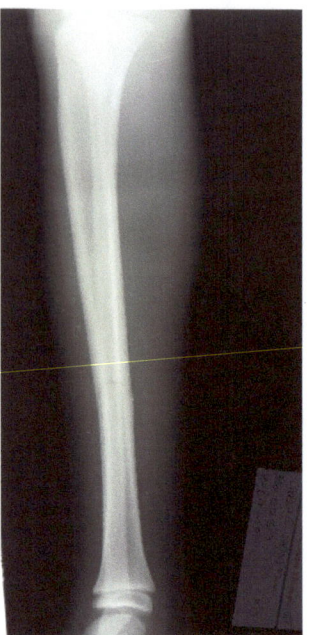

Radiograph – Lat. view: fracture tibia

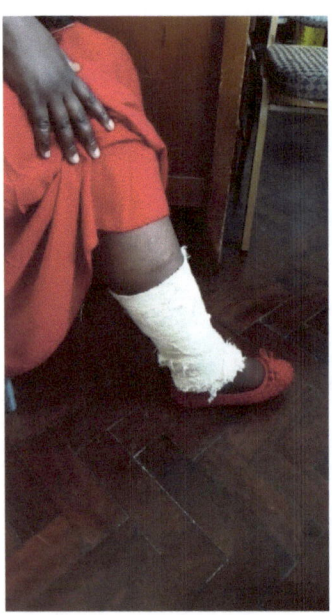

Picture 59A: Worn **former complete circular below knee POP**

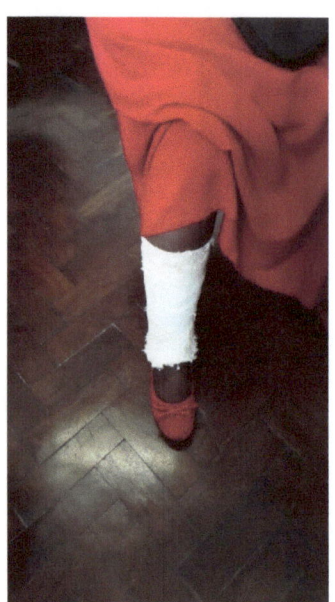

Picture 59B: A sign of a healed leg fracture

Note: A worn out "sole" of the POP foot (as shown above, both in children and adults) may be a sign of a healed fracture because the patient has been able to weight bear on the injured foot/leg

When a patient, child or adult, walks into your consultation room with a dirty and worn out POP, especially, on the sole of the foot, the fracture under that cast is most probably healed. If however the sole of the cast is as clean as you had applied it, it may mean that the fracture is not healed regardless of the empirical period of the limb being in the POP. A clinical assessment however must be done to establish whether or not the fracture is healed.

Again, the adjacent joint to the fracture may be developing some degree of stiffness. In that case, both for the upper and lower limbs, the patient must then be referred to the physiotherapy department so that the rehabilitation can be continued especially on the stiff or ensuing joint stiffness as regards the range of motion and strengthening exercises of the limb.

*M*aintenance of any "works" is important. In this regard, it is important to educate the patient on how to care for the plaster. These instructions can either by delivered to the patient verbally or on a small piece of paper – preferably well typed out. Some of the instructions are as follows:

1. Do not soak the limb (in POP) in water or any liquid

2. Do not sit near a fire (heat) with the POP in-situ (especially during the cold seasons of the year as the POP gets very hot and may burn the skin under the cast

3. If and when the POP feels or becomes loose, the patient should report back to the health facility for a check-up

4. When the POP is cracked, the patient must report back to the hospital

5. If the patient feels pain in an area which is away from the fracture site, the patient must report back to the health facility

6. If the patient's heel fails to reach the ground on walking due to a POP applied with a foot in equinus, the patient must report back to the health facility because this may lead to other complications like decubitus ulcers on the anterior aspects of the distal leg or the anterior ankle area.

7. If the POP feels tight, the patient must elevate the limb and move the toes or fingers whatever the case may be; if (s)he does not get any relief within 30 minutes to one hour, the patient must call back to the health facility

8. Patient must follow instructions as regards weight bearing; if the instructions are "non-weight bearing, partial weight bearing or full weight bearing, the patient should follow such instructions.

9. Use of crutches must also be explained. If the patient will use one crutch, it must be place on the contra-lateral (opposite side of the lower limb injury). This allows the patient to ambulate in a more near normal and natural way.

10. Do not bear weight on the lower limb 36 hours after the POP application to allow it to cure (harden effectively)

Note: As a medical staff in attendance, please learn to listen to the patient's symptoms when they do come back prior to the scheduled subsequent appointment date.

*I*t imperative that we do not just learn how to apply a good POP cast but rather invest time and resources, also, in learning how to safely remove the POP cast. There are a number of ways of removing the cast. The principles however remain the same; do not cause any harm.

From the onset, it must be mentioned that the electric POP cutter can cause injuries to the patient; it easily cuts the skin when not properly used; especially if and when applied with some degree of force or pressure! And because it a "noisy" power tool, it scares not only children but adults too. Children's skin is softer and delicate; it should therefore *NOT* to be used in children (especially in infants and toddlers).

The following are the tools (materials) that should be available for the removal of the POP

1. *Water*

2. *Manual POP shear*

3. *Power (electric) cutter and a tongue-depressor-like metal plate (spatula)*

4. *Spreader*

5. *A pair of POP scissors*

6. *Surgical blade – large size*

7. *Mat or Macintosh*

8. *Bucket*

Preparation

A good cook will always prepare the utensils and materials for her cooking. At the end of any procedure, the cook will have prepared the materials to use to clean her utensils and work-place before (s)he retires for the day.

In a similar fashion a good plaster "technician" must prepare and know which tools that (s)he would use for the removal of the POP cast from a patient's limb. This saves on time both for the patient and the medical staff, and allows for an efficient way of doing things.

Method

Water

Water is used to remove POP in children. The mother is allowed to soak the baby's POP (herself) for a while under the supervision of a health provider (who is knowledgeable in the technique). She then identifies where the plaster cast bandage ended and begins to unwind the wet bandage.

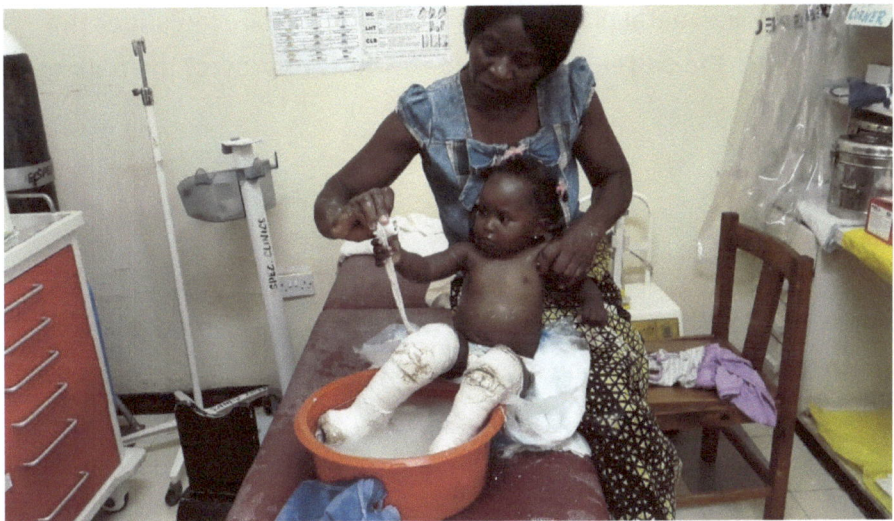

Picture 60: A mother removing (unwinding) a water-soaked POP bandage (it is comfortable for the child)

The Electric Cutter

The electric cutter and manual shear must be directed in anatomical areas that have more soft tissue; avoiding areas where there is subcutaneous bone e.g. along the ulna bone or the shin over the tibia; and pressure areas like the malleoli in the ankle area or the styloid processes in the wrist. Remember that the two cutting devices are best used on a thick, hard and well set POP. If the POP is soft or wet, the above two mentioned tools must not be used but a pair of scissors. A surgical blade must only be used with caution.

The electric cutter must not be used the way an electric rotating blade is used in cutting wood; sliding it from one end to the other. The electric saw oscillates about the center of the blade at a very fast speed. It is therefore advised that the oscillating blade is placed perpendicular to the POP surface (to be cut), and pressed gently through the thickness of the POP until a "give" is felt (this is into the under cast wool) and immediately withdrawn (to avoid injuring the skin). The blade is then withdrawn completely out of the cut area and placed to the end of the preceding cut. This is repeated from one end of the cast to the other (either from proximal to distal or vice versa); with a down-up, down-up maneuver.

As a precautionary measure, it is good practice to push a wooden or metallic tongue depressor between the skin and the intended area for cutting. The tongue depressor protects the skin from injury. *It must be noted that the electric cutter must be held at the roughened (neck) between the body and the oscillating blade as you press it into the POP to cut. The handler has better control of the tool than holding it by the body or tail of the electric cutter.*

a) Forearm POP

> The shear must be introduced on the palmar aspect of the hand and forearm and work upwards towards the elbow along the midline of the forearm. If an electric cutter is to be used, a tongue-depressor-like metal plate (spatula) must be introduced under the POP along the direction where the cutter will "traverse". This is to protect the patient's skin from injury.

b) Above elbow POP

> Just like above, the cutter follows the space between the cubital fossa and the lateral epicondyle and onto the lateral aspect of the arm.

c) Below Knee POP

> The POP may be cut following either the inner or outer margins of the foot. Starting from the toes and along the tough skin of the medial or later aspects of the foot; then proceed towards, below, around and behind the malleoli. Then proceed on the posterolateral or posteromedial aspects of the leg; avoiding any subcutaneous and superficial areas of bony parts. The reverse is also a safe route; by starting proximally and proceed distally tracing the above said route in the reverse direction.

Note1: An electric POP cutter must not be used on a child!!
Note2: For the purpose of this manual a surgical blade must not be used at all to remove the POP cast!!

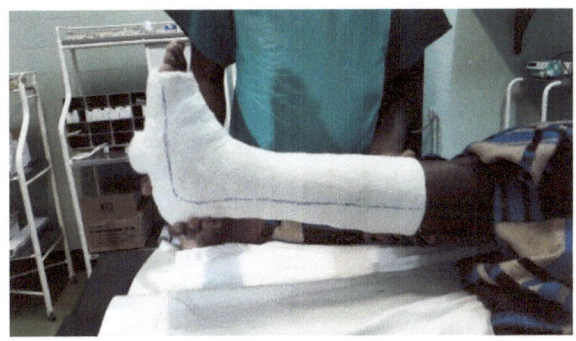 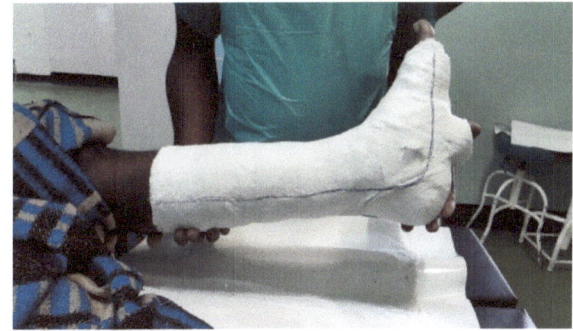

Picture 61A-B: Markings on the lateral and medial aspects of a Below Knee POP where a cut can be done using a manual shear or electric cutter for removal. Note: The markings go posterior to the medial and lateral malleoli (avoiding the bony prominences of malleoli)

d) Above Knee POP

Removing the above knee POP follows the same procedure as in the below knee POP except caution must be taken when maneuvering across the knee. Over the knee, the POP must be cut just lateral or medial to the patella (in the "hollow" parts of the knee); and then follow the any route above that (as the thigh is well padded with muscle). The lateral or medial aspects, however, are easier to run through.

The manual Shear

Note that there various types of POP shears. An example of a manual shear is shown in the *pictures 62A-B below:*

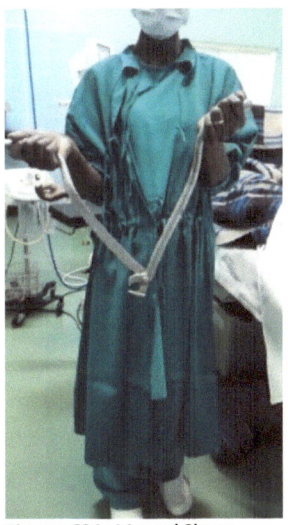 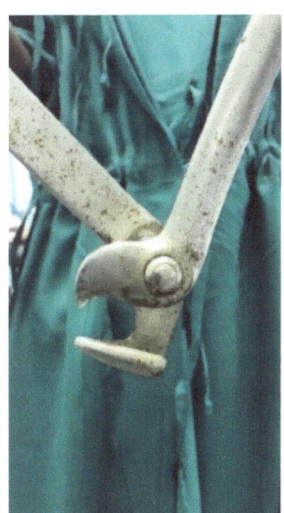

Picture 62A: Manual Shear **Picture 62B:** A close up of shear

The spreader has thicker "lips". It is therefore difficult for it to be introduced along the "cut off" line of the electric cutter. It is therefore advisable to create an oval "cut out" alongside the initial linear cut. The "island" so created is then removed using either a blunt point of the scissors or picked out with the index finger and the thumb. After this, the spreader is then introduced and split the POP along its length.

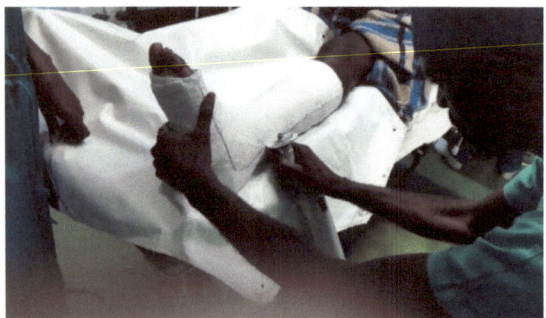

Picture 63A: Sequence of cutting the POP using the electric cutter Holding cutter by the roughened part (neck)

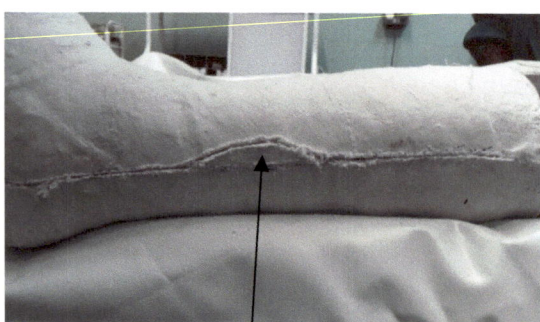

Picture 63B: Point at which to introduce a spreader

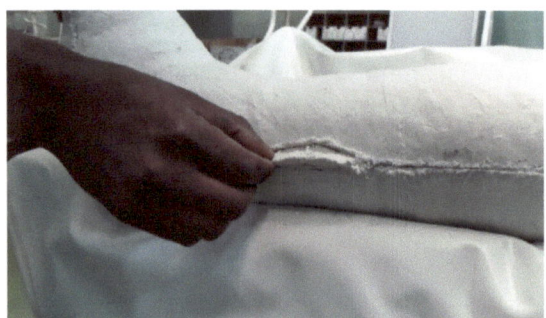

Pictures 63C: Picking the "island" piece out

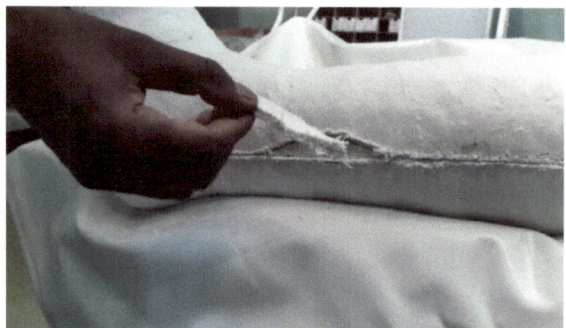

Picture 63D: Removal the "island" for the spreader

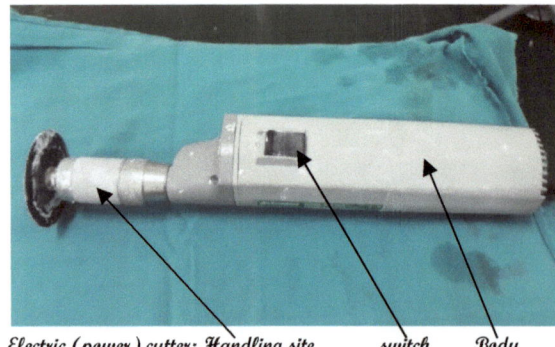

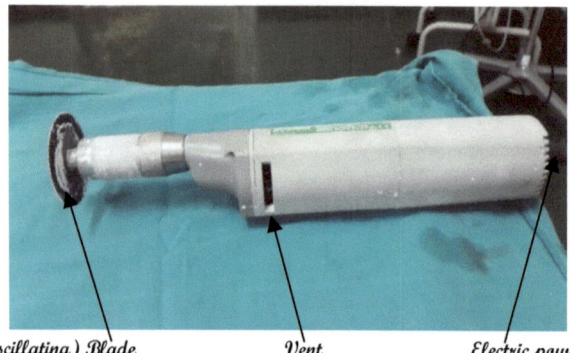

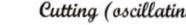

Electric (power) cutter: Handling site   switch   Body   Cutting (oscillating) Blade   Vent   Electric power cable

Picture 64A-B: Showing the parts of an electric POP cutter

This is a custom made type of scissors specifically for the use in the removing or cutting out POP. The lower lip had a longer, blunt and spatula like end. This is to make it safe from causing injury to the patient. If any other form of scissor is used, caution must be exercised. The pair of POP scissor is largely used to cut remnants of cotton from the POP plaster and the under-cast material.

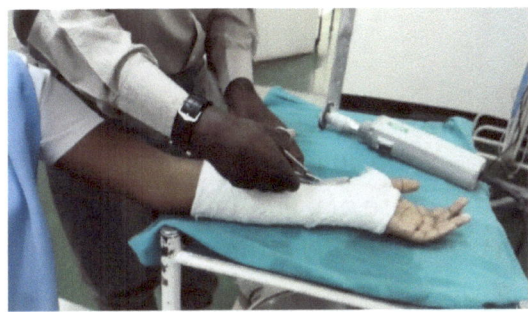

Pic 65A: Cutting the under cast with a scissors along midline from proximal to distal

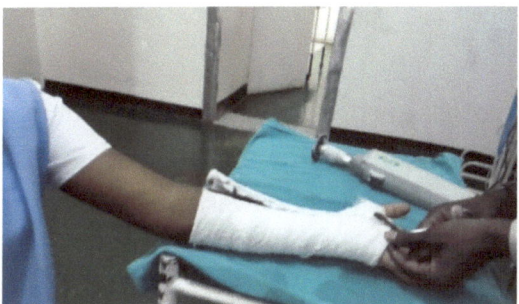

Picture 65B: Cutting the under cast from distal to proximal

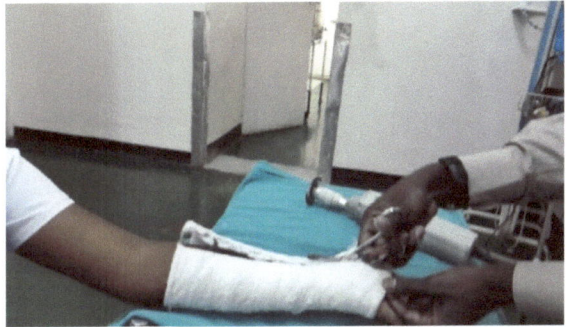

Picture 65C: Proximal cut meeting with the distal cut

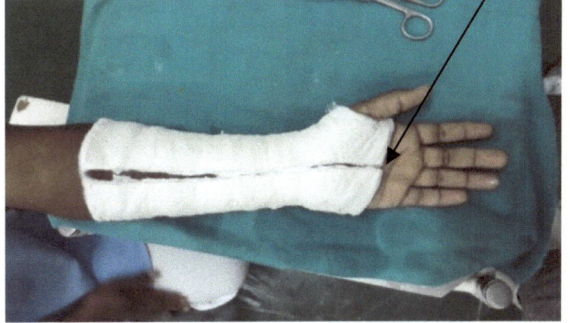

Clear distal palmar crease

Picture 65D: Complete cut along the midline ("fleshy area")

Use of a surgical Blade

The surgical blade can be used pretty much like the scissors. However extreme caution must be exercised. For the purpose of this manual, it must not be used.

After care

Nursing care

*a*ll patients with upper limb fractures and in a cast must go home (must be discharged) in some form of support. This can take the form of collar & cuff or arm-sling depending on the personality of the fracture. This gives the patient more relief and comfort as they travel back home.

Physiotherapy

Physiotherapy or physical therapy is an important component of non-operative fracture management. And as such, physiotherapy must be instituted as soon as is possible. The pain management of course takes precedence; however, physiotherapy must not be precluded because of pain. The pain must be managed actively while physiotherapy is underway. Even though the limb is under the cast physiotherapy can be and must be instituted; more so isometric exercises (for muscles under the cast) and active joint mobilization of joints outside the POP cast should be encouraged.

This is the reason why all the patients that are being discharged from the hospital must go through the physiotherapy department for advice and guidance.

Crutches and/or other walking aids will be prescribed appropriately. If or when a single crutch is to be used, the patient will be advised to use the crutch on the contralateral side (or opposite side) of the injured lower limb injury (as shown in the *picture 66A-B below*). The physiotherapist will drill the patient on how to use the appropriate walking aid.

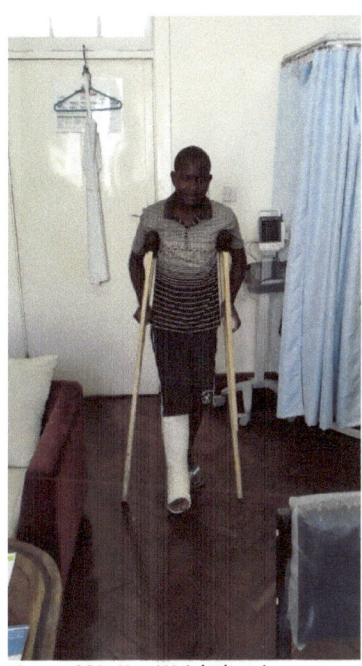

Picture 66A: Non Weight bearing

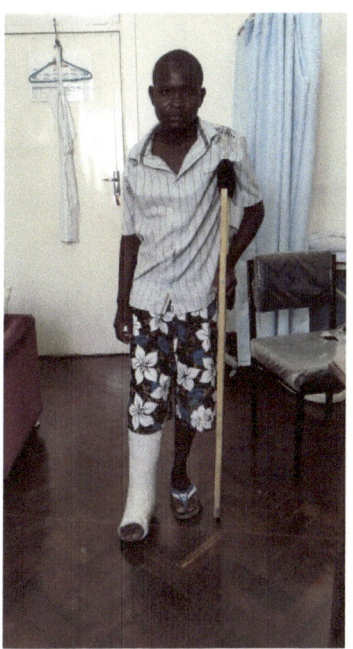

Picture 66B: Use of a crutch on the opposite side of injury

*I*t must be remembered that there are a number of complications that may occur due to injudicious and non-compliant ways of applying, using as well as caring for the POP cast. Some of these complications are:

1. Fracture blisters (see picture below)

2. Compartment syndrome

    a. Ischaemic contractures

    b. Loss of a limb (amputation) if the above said complication is not identified or recognized early

3. Decubitus ulcers (pressure sole) especially on pressure points plus secondary infection (soft or hard tissue) may follow.

4. Stiffness of the joints and contractures – due to prolong use of the POP – due to

    a. Surrounding tissues and

    b. Synovial membrane

5. Delayed union, non-union and mal-union of the fracture, osteoporosis

6. Soft injury (especially on removing the cast while using an electric cutter)

    a. Nerve damage

    b. Blood vessel damage

    c. Lymphatic tissue damage – chronic oedema

7. Muscle atrophy (this is a relative complication. However it is more pronounced in prolonged use of POP)

8. Damage to cartilage, forming pannus and ultimate degenerative joint disease

9. Ligamentous damage (shortening)

It is therefore important and imperative that the treatment of both the soft and the bone tissues are actively managed even when the appendage is under the cast so that the unnecessarily prolonged usage of Plaster of Paris is avoided and that the cast is removed at the shortest possible expected time!

Note: A complete circular below knee POP was applied on a freshly sustained close fracture resulting in fracture blisters; severe oedema (complications). This is not uncommon mistake and may result, unfortunately, into amputation of (an unfortunate) limb if left unchecked (pictures 68A-C)

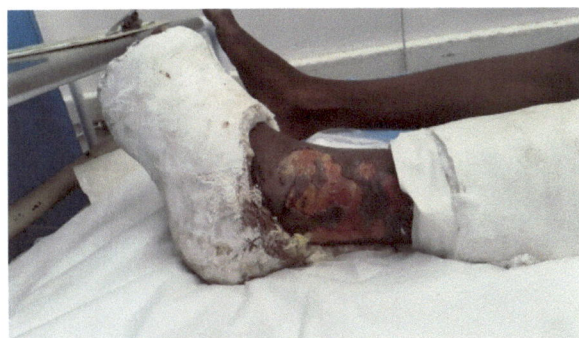

Picture 67A: Burst fracture blisters on the lateral aspect on a swollen leg

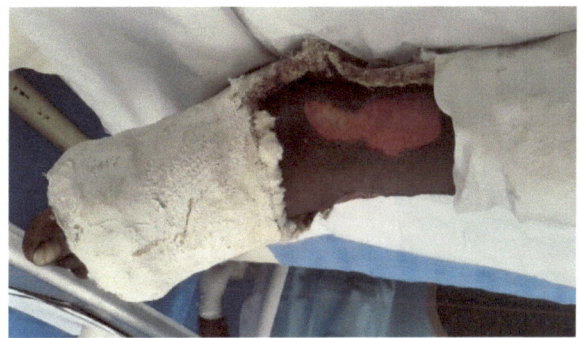

Picture 67B: Burst fracture Blister on the medial side on the distal leg

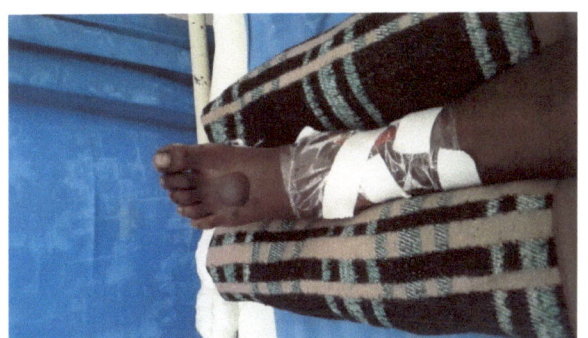

Picture 67C: Plaster of Paris is removed to actively manage the soft tissues

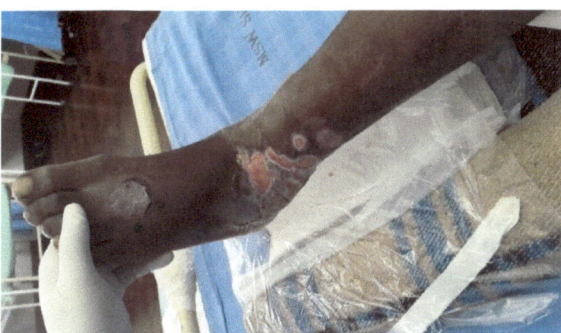

Picture 67D: One week following exposure

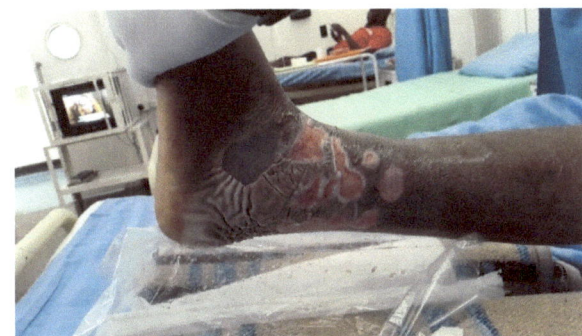

Picture 67E: Soft tissues healing (lateral) – one week later

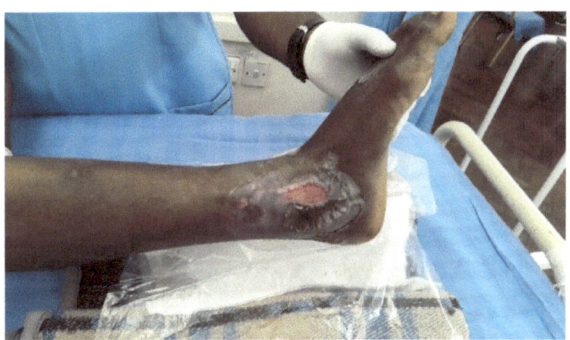

Picture 67F: Medial side – one week later

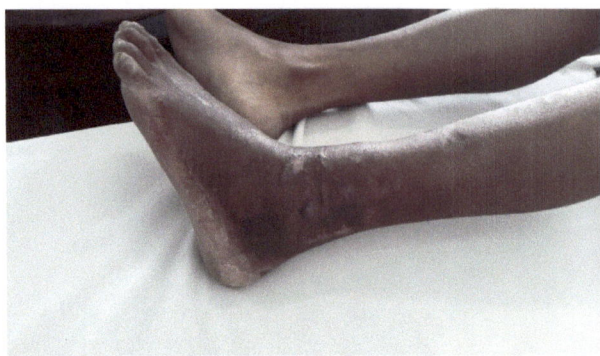
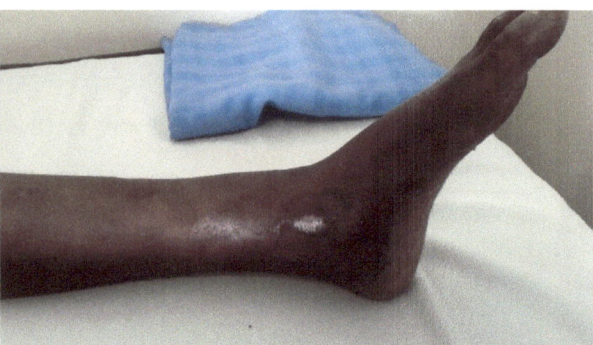

Picture 67G: Healed soft tissues (4 weeks post injury) – lateral side   **Picture 67H:** Medial side

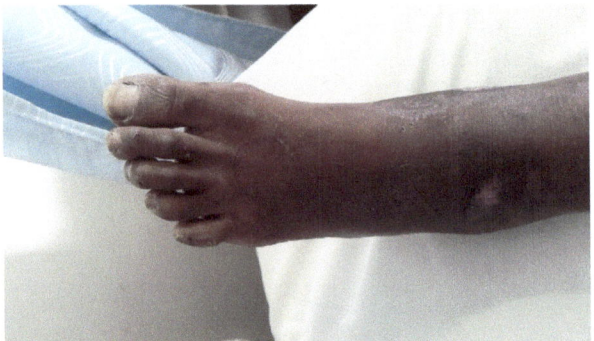

Picture 67I: Front (dorsal) aspect of the foot – 4 weeks post injury

Note that soft tissue management is important to the final fracture management!!!

References:

1. Apley's System of Orthopaedics and Fractures, 9[th]Ed by L Solomon, D Warwick, S Nayagam

2. A brief history of plaster and gypsum; www.infratechgypsum.com/gypsum_plaster.html

Shadrick G Lungu lives and works in Chingola, Zambia. He is married to Dr. Martha CM Lungu and between them have two lovely children, Dalitso (a boy) and Zamiwe, a girl.

He is a Senior Consultant Orthopaedic & Trauma Surgeon and a graduate of the University of Zambia. He was attached to Kalafong and Pretoria Academic Hospitals of the University of Pretoria, in the Republic of South Africa before graduating with a merit in Master of Surgery in Orthopaedics.

He has published a number of medical papers in various medical journals and is a Foundation Fellow of The College of Surgeons of East, Central & Southern Africa, a fellow in Spine Surgery from Assuit University, Egypt, a Charter member of the Institute of Arbitrators (London), holder of a Certificate in Business Administration.

He is an honorary lecturer for AO/ASIF Foundation; an organization striving to improve Orthopaedic and trauma care for/of the patients in the economically challenged countries of the world. He is an honorary member of the SADC group of Prosthetics and Orthotics since May 2015.

He belongs to two service and charitable organizations respectively. He is a Progressive Melvin Jones Fellow of the Associations of Lions Clubs International and District Governor for District 413 Zambia for the year 2015-2016 and Deputy Chairperson for Mission Medic Air, respectively.

His hobbies are reading, writing (and doing research) watching documentaries on Digital Satellite Television where old dead classic cars are transformed into "new" ones, football and boxing. He also loves listening to Jazz and Blues...

Other projects under way are semi-fictional novels; the titles are "My Past Started Yesterday"; "When I Lost My Twin..." and "The Treasure on The Sweet Island"

He gets his inspiration from his work as a doctor, books of other writers and from his worldwide travels.

It is therefore his sincere hope and trusts that the general readership, worldwide, will find this book to be of great value to deliver a systematic and sustainable service to the students and more importantly the end user, the patient.

Index

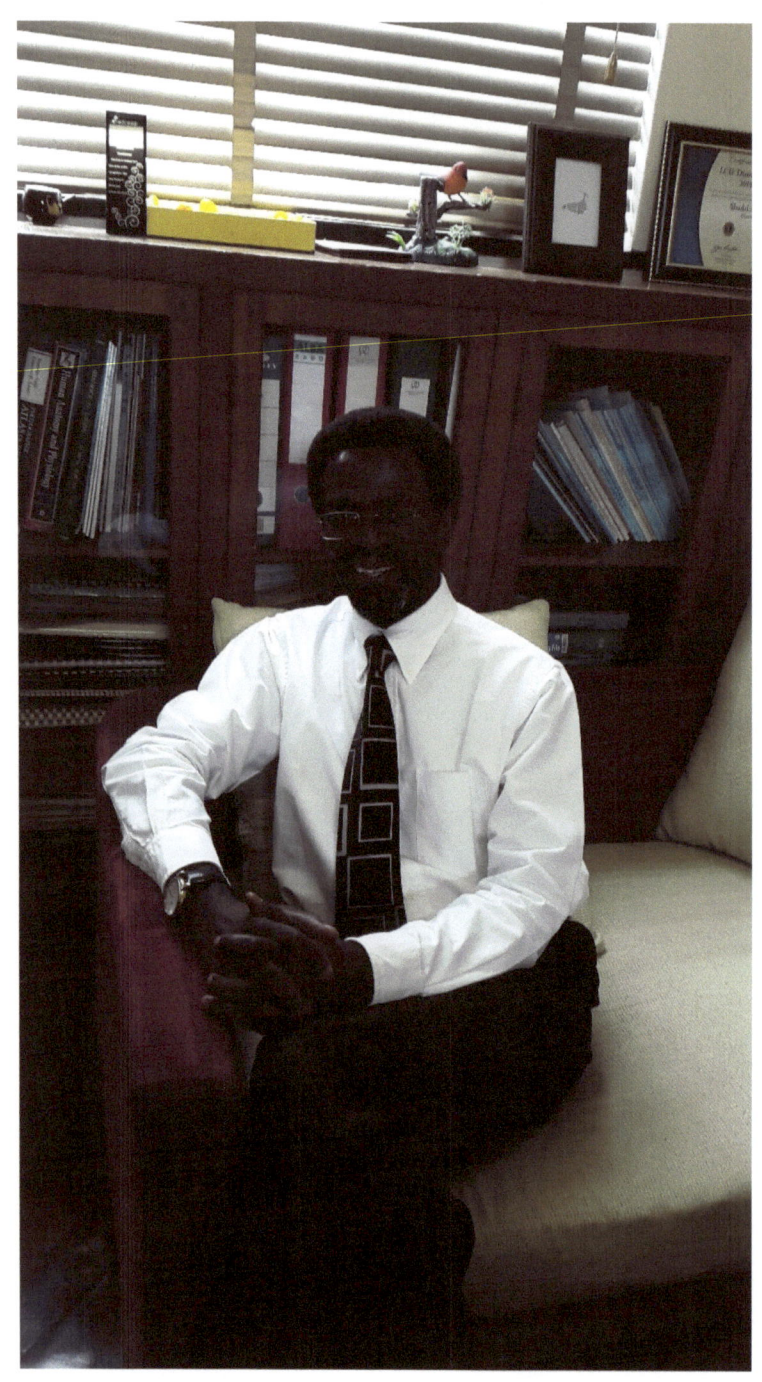

Notes...

Notes...

Notes...

Notes...

Notes...

Notes...

www.ingramcontent.com/pod-product-compliance
Lightning Source LLC
Chambersburg PA
CBHW050718180526
45159CB00003B/1064